THINGS NOBODY KNOWS BUT ME

THINGS NOBODY KNOWS BUT ME

AMRA PAJALIĆ

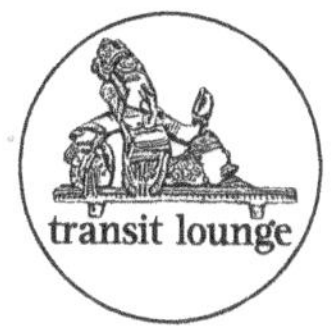

MELBOURNE, AUSTRALIA
www.transitlounge.com.au

First published 2019
Transit Lounge Publishing

Cover image: Glasshouse Images / Alamy Stock Photo
Cover and book design: Peter Lo

Printed in Australia by McPherson's Printing Group

Pre-publication data is available from the
National Library of Australia: trove.nla.gov.au
ISBN: 978-1-925760-20-0

Dedicated to my mother, Fatima, and all the women who came before me whose lives were full of sacrifice, so that mine could be full of choices. And for my daughter, Sofia, who stands on the shoulders of these strong women and is able to reach for the sky because of them.

AUTHOR'S NOTE

This is my story, but more than that it is my mother's story. I have changed names in order to protect the anonymity of some people, and in some instances I have also changed identifying details.

In writing this book I have used my notebooks, journals and diaries, medical records obtained through Freedom of Information requests, research undertaken at the State Library of newspaper articles, interviews of my family and my own (possibly fallible) memory.

As such, while every event depicted in this book did occur, I have used fictional devices to recreate dialogue and setting. In some instances I have also compressed timelines slightly in order to create narrative flow.

PROLOGUE

I was sixteen when my wagging caught up to me. It started when I stayed home to ensure my mother didn't drive while she was under the influence of her illness, but I continued to forge her signature long after she recovered.

I ended up in my high school counsellor's office. 'Mum has nervous breakdowns,' I told Miss Meadowcroft.

She frowned. 'What does she suffer from?'

'What do you mean?' Mum called it *Slom Živaca* in Bosnian, which translated to 'nervous breakdown' in English. That's what she and everyone I knew called it, and that's what I'd grown up telling people.

Miss Meadowcroft asked me what happened when Mum got sick. I explained how she got insomnia and cleaned the walls with bleach until her hands were pruned and wrinkled. That she went on shopping sprees at Copperart and emptied our bank account. The way she physically transformed, with her green eyes glowing as if she were drug-affected, and her speech slurring as if her tongue were too thick in her mouth. The delusions that spewed from her lips: that she was going to speak to the President of the United States and stop wars, or that she was training to race an Olympic champion.

Miss Meadowcroft nodded as I spoke.

I explained that there was no logic to Mum getting sick.

She got sick when she was taking her medication, sometimes she got sick when she didn't. She got sick when she was stressed, and she got sick when she wasn't. The one thing that was a constant was the complete shock I felt every time. It seemed as if her illness transformed her overnight from a caring mother to a self-involved woman who was unaware of anyone else.

Miss Meadowcroft's questions made me think. I went home that night and asked Mum what her illness was called.

'Nervous breakdown.'

'What causes it?'

'The doctors told me that there was a chemical imbalance in the brain.'

I was bewildered. This was the first time I'd thought of her illness as something that could be controlled.

When I returned the next time to talk to Miss Meadowcroft she had a surprise for me.

'I did some research about your mum.' She handed me some sheets of paper that were photocopied pages from a book. 'Does this sound like your Mum's illness?'

I took the sheets and began reading. The sheets were about manic depression and described it as an illness that was characterised by manic highs and depressive lows. When the person was suffering from mania they engaged in impetuous and reckless behaviour, including spending money, being sexual and losing inhibitions. When they suffered from lows they would struggle to get out of bed and become suicidal. (More recently the illness has become known as bipolar disorder.)

As I read I felt a shock thrumming through my system. I didn't know it at the time, but this moment would change my life.

'This is my mum,' I gasped. There was a pattern to my mother's illness. It wasn't something that just happened, but instead there were signs that until this point I had been ignorant about.

I went home with the pieces of paper. 'Mum, I think you have manic depression.'

Mum looked at me with curiosity. 'Some doctors said I have schizophrenia, some said manic depression.'

'This is all about you.' I handed her the pieces of paper.

She took them from me and read.

'This is what you have, isn't it?' I asked.

Mum nodded.

'Why did you call it nervous breakdown?'

'That's what we called it at home.'

My mother's homeland was Bosnia, once called Yugoslavia, which used to be under Communist rule. Mental illness was stigmatised and shameful. This had shaped her view of her illness as an affliction and a curse. Her rudimentary English also made it difficult for her to engage in the medical jargon surrounding her illness.

After this, everything changed. It was like a veil had been ripped away from my eyes: I stopped seeing Mum's illness as an entity that had no logic. Having the correct label meant understanding that Mum had no control when she was under the influence of her illness. Until then I had judged her and found her wanting: as a mother, a wife, a human being. I realised I couldn't judge Mum for her failings. She was a victim of her own brain chemistry, and as her daughter my role was to accept and love her for who she was, not who I wanted her to be.

This is our story.

PART I

A DIFFERENT KIND OF MUM

When I was four years old I watched my mum climb the stairway to heaven and wondered what she would find when she got up there. Would she see God or would she just fall back to earth?

It had all started a few weeks earlier. While Mum had always been religious, now her fervour became all-consuming until she was convinced that God was communicating with her.

I was in the backyard with my two-year-old brother. We were sitting in the leftover sand from one of my father's many do-it-yourself projects, making shapes with plastic containers and water, while Mum hung out the washing. Mum suddenly stopped and cocked her head as if she was listening to someone. She dropped the sheet in her hands and approached the tall shelves my father had built to store his tools, which ran up the wall of the house and reached the roof. Mum looked like an angel in her long, flowing dress, her brown hair a halo.

'Yes, Allah, I know you are looking after me and I will prove it to everyone,' Mum said to God. She closed her eyes as she took her first step, climbing the shelf as if it was a ladder. '*Bismillah, ir-Rahman, ir-Rahim.*' *In the name of God, the Most Gracious, the Most Merciful*, she prayed in Arabic, the shared language of all Muslim prayers, as she climbed.

My mother had told me that God was all-knowing, all-seeing, but that he had no shape or body. I didn't know where to send my prayers and so I watched mutely, terrified of Mum falling or the untethered shelves falling on her, as I waited for God to reveal himself.

Mum reached the top and paused as her hands touched the roof tiles. She stopped, her dress billowing in the faint summer breeze, before she climbed back down slowly, her eyes still firmly closed. '*Allahu Ekber*,' she repeated over and over, '*Allahu Ekber*,' praising God. 'See, I told you God would protect me.'

While I accepted my mother's words as a fact, I also realised she was different to the other mothers in the Bosnian community. Other mothers spent their days cooking and cleaning, always on the move as they cared for their family. My mother would bundle us into the car and take us visiting, staying for hours and not returning until dark, when she would perform the household chores she had neglected. When the mania of bipolar disrupted her sleep, she would vacuum late at night, while my brother and I sat sleepily on the couch waiting to go to bed. Or she would cook in the early hours of the morning, the sound of clanging pots floating into the edges of my dreams, the aroma of fresh bread filling the house.

That night my mother's voice woke me from a deep sleep. Sitting up in bed, I saw a bright light under the door. I lay back down and my brother curled up against me. Since Dad went away we all slept together in the bed Mum had shared with him. My brother and I couldn't sleep alone, waking up and searching out Mum during the night, and so she'd started lying down with us at bedtime. I hadn't realised she would get up again after we were asleep.

I closed my eyes but now it seemed the shadows around the bed were full of menace, making me tighten with fear. I gently eased myself out of bed so I didn't wake my brother and opened the bedroom door. Mum was sitting in the hallway, her back against the wall next to the bedroom, the phone in her lap. The phone cord in the hallway limited her ability to move around. There was an ashtray next her, and smoke clouds hung in the air. Later I learnt that she was talking to Lifeline counsellors.

'I feel like it's my fault,' she said. 'I wished that he would die and then it came true.'

'Mummy, what are you doing?' I asked, rubbing the tears from my eyes.

Mum quickly hung up the phone.

'I was scared,' I said.

Mum took me back to the bedroom and once again we lay side by side until I fell asleep. Her voice on the phone woke me again, but fatigue eventually tipped me back into sleep.

Over the next few weeks Mum slept less and less, and she began spending every night on the phone. I learnt to sleep through her one-sided conversations, comforting myself that she was just outside the bedroom door and the monsters couldn't find us.

A few nights later Mum woke us up. She was sitting on the bed and the light spilling into the darkened room from the hallway behind her made her look like a shadow looming over us. Usually she was trying to get us to fall asleep or stay asleep so she could maintain her nocturnal habits, and I was scared at the change in her priorities.

'You and your brother need to pray for Babo,' she said, the words jumping off her tongue like machine-gun bullets. 'Allah will value the prayers from a child much higher and your Babo will go to heaven. Now, repeat after me.' Her green eyes glowed as she recited the Arabic prayer. '*Bismilahi Irahman Irahim* –'

We repeated the prayer until my eyes were too heavy and I couldn't keep them open anymore. Over the next few weeks we prayed together every night until I learnt to do it myself. This became my nightly ritual and for years I couldn't fall asleep until I had said my prayer, sending my father a blessing in heaven.

The next day there was a knock on the door. When Mum opened it, a man in a black robe and a white turban crossed the threshold. I had seen those clothes when we went to the mosque and knew this man was the *Hodža*, a Bosnian imam. I was surprised to see him, as he had never visited our house before.

'*Salam Alejkum.*' Mum greeted him with the Arabic phrase that meant 'peace be upon you'.

'*Alejkumu Salam,*' the *Hodža* replied.

Mum led the *Hodža* to the kitchen, and my brother and I followed. They sat across from each other at the kitchen table.

'How can I help you, my sister?' the *Hodža* asked as he fixed his gaze on Mum.

'I can't sleep at night. I'm restless and unsettled. I think there is a spirit in the house. I think my husband is haunting me,' Mum whispered to the *Hodža* as she looked at the kitchen wall.

My parents had moved into the house – a1950s-built, yellow-brick, three-bedroom house on a quarter-acre block – when they got married five years before. Like most migrants, my parents were looking to replicate their homeland in some way. The suburb of St Albans, in the western suburbs of Melbourne, became a Balkan enclave. Our neighbours were from Macedonia, Croatia, Serbia, Bosnia, Slovenija – all former republics that formed the country that was then called Yugoslavia.

The day my mother's guilt was born was etched in her memory, and like a movie she replayed it over and over in the years to come. My mother told me that she was washing the dishes while my father sat at the kitchen table behind her. She finished the last dish and soaked her hands in the sudsy water, not wanting to turn around and look at him. He'd found her that morning in the shower, beating her head against the tiles as she cried, her throat producing raw screams of rage and pain as the warm water soothed her bruised body. In five years of marriage, his slaps and punches had left bruises like a rubber stamp on her body. She had attempted to leave him but had been terrified of becoming a two-time divorcee before she turned thirty, and so she stayed.

My father had suffered from stomach pains for years and took fistfuls of Panadol throughout the day. Eventually the pain wore him down and he went to a doctor, who began tests. She had served him coffee when he returned from the doctor's appointment, before going to the sink to wash the dishes. She knew he wanted her to ask him what happened, but she wouldn't give him that satisfaction.

'The doctors think I have cancer,' my father finally said.

'Did you hear me?' he asked, his voice breaking on the last word. 'The doctors think I have cancer and that I'm going to die.'

Mum lifted her hands from the sink and wiped them on a tea towel. She turned around and walked past him. As her hand turned the doorknob on the back door she thought to herself, *I couldn't be that lucky*, and went outside.

They didn't speak about it again. He underwent surgery but as soon as they opened him up they saw that the pancreatic cancer was too advanced.

The five-year survival rate upon diagnosis of pancreatic cancer was then 5 per cent. It was assumed that the cancer was terminal because it was so aggressive and it was generally only discovered when it was too late, but over the years doctors have realised the opposite. It has such a high incidence of mortality because it is so slow and insidious in its advancement and is usually only discovered when it has decimated the pancreas. The cause of the cancer was unknown, but it seems that smokers and drinkers of alcohol are at higher risk and my father had adopted both vices at twelve years old. He used to sell his textbooks for alcohol, spending the day in the woods getting drunk and committing mischief.

Mum was in the waiting room when the doctor came to see her after the surgery. 'I'm afraid we have bad news. Hasim's cancer is too advanced for us to remove the cancer surgically. We believe he will only live six months to a year.'

Mum swayed under the weight of his words.

'He is still under anaesthetic, but we'll tell him when he wakes.'

'Do you have to?' Mum asked. 'Maybe it's better that he doesn't know.'

In the old country doctors kept a terminal prognosis to themselves. They thought it was cruel to tell a patient that they were dying when there was nothing to be done. Instead they recommended that the patient went to a spa to restore their health, thus giving them the opportunity to get some hard-wrung enjoyment in their last moments.

'I'm sorry,' the doctor said. 'We have a legal obligation to let our patients know about their prognosis.'

Mum nodded.

'I'll take you through.'

The doctor led her into my father's room. She sat on the chair and watched him as he slept. It didn't seem possible that he had only a year to live. His cheeks were pink and he looked in robust health. She would have thought the doctors were wrong if she didn't remember the way his face turned pale and his body contorted from pain as the cancer ate him from the inside.

When my father woke the doctor told him the prognosis. Mum watched his face and saw he wasn't surprised, but when the doctor left his eyes welled up.

'I'm not going to see them grow up,' he said. He started sobbing, deep gut-wrenching sobs of grief. I was four years old, my brother two.

Mum leaned forward and held his head against her chest as he cried. Her eyes were dry. She felt a coldness seep into her body. She'd wished him dead so many times and now it seemed that her wish was coming true.

The doctor told him that if he received chemotherapy treatment it would give him a better chance of living longer. He received two treatments, but his body did not tolerate the drugs and he felt so ill he wished for death. He chose a shorter life of quality; the doctors predicted that he had six months to live. He was thirty years old.

There was a scrics of photos in the album featuring him with friends, mementos of a dying man. There was a photo I was haunted by as a child and I took it to school for show-and-tell about special photos, hanging it up next to my classmates' holiday snaps and pictures of birthday fun. In the photo my father is sitting on the couch, his shirt unbuttoned, his best friend sitting next to him as they both stare unsmiling into the camera. They had been smoking and drinking, beer bottles and a full ashtray on the coffee table in front of them.

My father's eyes looked haunted, as if he was seeing something behind the camera that terrified him. As an adult I imagined that this was the moment he decided to stop the chemotherapy and face a certain death. As a child I was devastated that the other children laughed when I pinned the photograph to the noticeboard. All they saw was a man in his underwear sitting on the couch, whereas all I could see was his sorrow. When I returned from recess they had moved the drawing pin holding the photo so that it was on his penis. I quietly removed the pin and returned the photo back the photo album, never to be put on display again.

Now as my mother poured out her fears to the *Hodža*, she hoped that he would absolve her of her guilt at wishing for my father's death.

'A spirit is afraid of Allah's prayer.' The *Hodža* took out two plastic bottles from his backpack. 'Fill these with water.' He got paper and a pen and began writing the Al-Fatihah, the first chapter of the Qur'an and a prayer for God's guidance, while Mum filled the bottles and placed them on the kitchen table between them.

The *Hodža* finished writing and folded the paper into a small triangle. He forced the paper through the top of a bottle and stood up. 'We will now chase away this spirit.'

My brother and I followed Mum and the *Hodža* into each of the rooms. He prayed loudly as he poured water onto his hand and sprinkled it onto the bed, the bedside tables, the floor, the windows. When he finished we returned to the kitchen and he handed the second bottle to Mum.

What the *Hodža* was practising was as far from religion as you could get. The Qur'an specifically forbids anything that is related to superstition and contains no such rituals to deal with spirits, but like most bereaved, my mother was vulnerable to fraudsters chasing their own gains.

'Drink this three times a day, my sister,' the *Hodža* said. 'Each time you drink, recite the Al-Fatihah prayer.'

Mum nodded and handed him money. He counted the notes and put them in his pocket. After we walked the *Hodža* out, I returned to my bedroom and rubbed my fingers in the water puddled on my bedside table. I lifted my fingers to my lips and tasted it. It didn't taste any different to tap water. Tiny fragments of paper stuck to my tongue like fur. That night my mother felt comforted by the *Hodža*'s ritual and did not seek the guidance of the Lifeline counsellors, but this empty ritual did not chase away her demons.

A few days later we heard a car pulling up in the driveway and Mum went to the window. My brother and I followed.

I stood on my tiptoes so I could see outside while Haris held onto my arm. Aida and her husband Zlatan were parked in the driveway. They were long-time family friends who had known my mother since she was a fifteen-year-old bride and a newly arrived migrant. When she had her first breakdown in hospital after giving birth at sixteen, they were the ones who visited her every day. They became her surrogate parents, since her own parents were on the other side of the world.

Mum opened the door. Our visitors took off their shoes and left them in the hallway, a custom that all Bosnians followed.

'Now go to the bathroom and perform your ablutions,' Mum ordered. Muslims had to cleanse themselves before commencing prayers.

My mother had started calling our house a mosque since the *Hodža* blessed the house. I had accepted her words and believed that we were blessed because God could hear us, and had started praying for him to grant me the ability to fly. But now as I watched Zlatan and Aida exchange confused glances, I realised that perhaps my mother was wrong and I would never get my wings.

'That's okay, we don't need to pray,' Aida finally said.

Mum, like her friends, was a cultural Muslim. She went to the mosque to pray on religious holidays, but she didn't perform the Muslim requirement of five prayers a day.

'You have to perform your ablutions when you come into a mosque,' Mum said.

'This isn't a mosque,' Aida said.

'Yes, it is.' Mum lifted her hands to encompass the walls around us. 'A *Hodža* blessed this house and made it a mosque.'

'Fatima, let's go to the living room and talk.' Aida took

Mum's hand and led her sit down. Aida and Zlatan sat on the couch, while Mum paced before them.

'We are worried about you,' Aida said.

'Why?' Mum demanded. 'I'm fine. Allah is protecting me.'

'Did you sleep at all?'

'I don't need to sleep. Allah is working through me and I am not a mortal any longer.'

Aida hesitated. She looked at her husband, but he just shifted uncomfortably and shrugged his shoulders. 'You need to see a doctor. You're scaring your children,' he said.

She looked at us. I wasn't scared up until this point, but now I wondered if I should be.

'Amra and Haris are fine. Allah has blessed this house and they are safe here,' Mum said, looking at my brother and me.

'You need to see a doctor,' Aida pleaded. 'You're not well, can't you see that?'

'I am fine.' Mum's voice was raised. 'I have no need of doctors. All I need to do is pray and I will be saved.' She raised her hands beside her head and said '*Allahu Akbar*,' which meant God is Great and was the preface to prayer. She folded her hands over her chest and began reciting verses of the Qur'an.

Aida tried to interrupt her but Mum continued praying. She was bowing three times, saying '*Subhana rabbiyal adheem*': God hears those who call upon Him; Our Lord, praise be to You.

'Fatima, we're going to have to call the hospital and take Amra and Haris into care.'

Mum stopped praying, these words acting like a slap to the face. 'No, please don't do that. Don't take them away. I just need to sleep.'

Mum had already had three instances of what she called *Slom Živaca* (which translated to 'nervous breakdowns'), each time after giving birth: first to my half-sister, then me and finally my brother. When she was hospitalised after birthing my brother my father had been home to care for me, but now we only had her.

Mum rubbed her eyes. 'I haven't slept for a long time.'

Aida led her to the couch and they spoke. Aida brought Mum's medication and she took her pills. After Mum managed to convince them that she would sleep that night and that this would calm her, they finally left.

My mother and her friends did not understand the symptomology of Mum's illness, and they believed that one good night of sleep and her regular dose of medication would solve it. What she really needed was a circuit breaker in the form of mood stabilisers.

When Aida and Zlatan returned the next day, Hava and Alija, the couple who rented the bungalow in our backyard, told them about Mum's strange behaviour during the night. In the early hours of the morning, they had woken up to the sound of Mum in the front yard shouting prayers in the rain, praising Allah. My brother and I had been asleep, unaware of her nocturnal outing.

Mum watched through the window as the two couples talked, her face creased with concern as she prayed in a whisper. Hava and Alija left and Aida and Zlatan headed for the front door.

They knocked, but Mum stood in the hallway, unmoving. She saw them as conspiring against her. They wanted to steal her children.

'Please, Fatima, open the door,' they pleaded as they knocked.

'Go away,' she shouted. 'There's nothing wrong with me.' She knew that once they entered the house she'd be admitted to hospital and my brother and I would be removed from her care.

At least an hour passed before Mum peered out the window and gasped. I went to stand beside her and looked outside. Two officers were getting out of a police car to speak with her concerned friends.

'Now they're using the police to steal you,' Mum said. She took hold of our hands and walked with us to the spare bedroom and locked the door.

There was a crash as the police smashed open the front door and the sound of footsteps as they entered.

'Fatima, open up.' Aida knocked on the bedroom door. 'You're scaring the children.'

Mum hugged my brother and me closer. 'You're not scared?'

'No,' I lied, and Haris repeated it after me. I believed that they wanted to steal us, and I hugged Mum tighter.

'You know Mum would never hurt you,' she said, staring straight ahead.

Aida kept shouting and knocking, then there was silence. A few minutes later came the sound of metal on metal and the handle started turning. The door handle was a simple one: all you needed to unlock it from the other side was a butter knife.

Aida unlocked the door and came in, heading towards me. Mum stood and rushed at her, a lioness protecting her cubs from those who meant them harm. They grappled, each of them pushing in the opposite direction. Mum's mental illness gave her super strength and with one strong push she heaved Aida out of the room and locked the door again.

We sat in the room for a long time. The two police officers appeared at the side of the house, their heads and shoulders visible in the window. They peered inside to see if Mum was hurting us. We sat still under their scrutiny. After exchanging a few words, they moved on.

'Fatima, this is Constable Reynolds. Please open the door.'

Mum kept praying under her breath. Again, there was the sound of someone picking the lock and the knob turned. The police officer entered, but Mum didn't move from the bed. He took her by the arm and gently led her out. 'Come, Fatima, we're taking you to the hospital.'

Mum went with the police officers compliantly. She was subdued by their male presence. She had been taught that men were aggressors and to protect herself she had to be meek and still. She looked like a small girl between the two brawny officers as they each held onto an arm and took her out of the house.

Aida rushed in. 'Are you all right?' She hugged Haris and me.

Years later I spoke to Mum about the incident. She shook her head and her face took on a bitter twist. 'They were acting like I was going to hurt you, but I would never hurt my child.'

And while I remembered feeling confused and frightened, I had never been scared of my own mother hurting me. It was only when I received her medical records under freedom of information that I truly understood what had happened.

The Footscray Psychiatric Hospital admission form states that Mum was admitted on 1 December 1982 after a referral by the Law Enforcement Agency. An informant told the police that she had locked herself in with her children and was praying and had threatened to kill her children. The neighbours told the admitting doctor that she was pinching her children with scissors.

I was startled. Had I blocked this out? But something didn't feel right. I had spent a whole lifetime with my mother and her mental illness. While she had threatened to take her own life, she had never once physically hurt me or Haris or anyone else.

I wonder whether my mother's friends, when faced with my mother's intractable refusal to go to hospital, had called the police to help. When the police officers arrived perhaps they had said they could only intervene if there was a possibility of harm and so my mother's friends had made claims that would ensure my mother would be admitted to hospital and my brother and I would be taken into care.

Years later I spoke to other children parented by bipolar sufferers. One of the women I met would be left alone with her sister for days without food when her mother disappeared. I had never experienced that kind of hardship. I always had shelter and food, and this was because of family friends who stepped up and took care of us, regardless of how they had to do it.

After Mum was admitted to hospital Haris and I went to live with Aida and Zlatan. The car pulled up in front of a double-storey house with large arched windows. They were extremely well-off and although they had no children their house was large and spacious – so different from our small, cramped home.

Later that day visitors arrived. Aida pulled us aside and told me that we weren't to eat any of the food that she served to visitors as that was rude. We had never heard of this rule. Whenever we had visitors we ate whatever they ate.

While we were playing one of our visitors looked over at us and shook her head sadly. 'They are like orphans, poor children. Their father is dead and their mother is a mental patient. At least there are good people like you to help them.' The visitor patted Aida's hand.

This was something I would hear repeated throughout my childhood. We were pitied because our mother was seen as inadequate by the standards of the Bosnian community.

We would visit Mum in hospital, each time feeling heartbroken and bereft when we had leave her behind and go back to our temporary home.

After a few months Mum was released and we were returned to her care. Once again we took turns sleeping next to her in bed and every night she would tell us the story of Baba Jaga, the Slavic version of the wicked witch who lived in the woods, but in my mother's stories she was a benevolent enchantress who tested the character of those she met and anointed the deserving with magical powers.

The medication made Mum lethargic and she slept late, sometimes until midday. While she slept my brother and I entertained ourselves. One day we pulled apart the L-shaped lounge suite and every section was a different country. Another game was transforming the lush mulberry tree in our backyard into a cubby house by placing cardboard boxes on the branches and our toys in each room. When summer came and the berries ripened the toys stayed in the tree and became permanently stained from the fruit.

Alija and Hava lived in the bungalow behind our house.

They were a remnant of Mum's life with my father. Even though they were tenants, they soon behaved like my grandparents. In a life of chaos, they provided some much needed stability and boundaries.

One morning I was making toast while Mum slept. The toaster didn't have an automatic timer to eject the toast. I was watching cartoons and lost track of time. It was only when I smelt something burning that I remembered. I ran to the kitchen. The bread was on fire; flames lit up the orange toaster. I shrieked in panic. I remembered what firefighters did and got a tea towel and tried to smother the flames. The tea towel caught fire and sparks spread across the kitchen table.

I saw Hava through the back flyscreen door. She'd probably smelt the fire and heard my shrieks. I knew that if she saw what had happened I would get in trouble, and so would Mum. 'Close the door,' I yelled. Haris obeyed and shut the door with a bang.

The fire was still burning. I ran to the sink and got a glass of water, throwing it onto the toaster.

The fire was gone. So was the electricity.

We became untamed children under my mother's lax parental control, with no bedtime routine and no rules. My brother and I only had each other and it was our job to protect Mum from well-meaning adults who saw her as an adult-child incapable of performing her parental responsibilities.

Our mother was different, but that's what we liked about her. While other children had strict routines and consequences, we had freedom and frivolity – and we didn't want the party to end.

GAME

I knelt over the coffee table, drawing squiggly circles on a lined notepad. My brother sat across from me, playing with his toy truck. I tore out the finished page and carelessly threw it on the pile of circle-filled sheets lying on the floor beside me.

I looked through the kitchen doorway and saw Mum talking to her friend Anisa. They were sitting at opposite sides of the dining table, each holding a *fildžan* cup in one hand and clutching a cigarette in the other. They alternated between lifting the cigarette to suck at the filter, and lifting the cup to sip hot coffee.

The kitchen window reflected their silhouettes against the backdrop of black night. A blue haze of cigarette smoke rose over them like a mist, creeping up to the ceiling and through the rest of the flat, the stale smell seeping into furniture and clothing.

I looked back at the paper, drawing ever wider circles to fill the lines. I sensed movement and looked up. Anisa's son Fadil had entered the living room. He knelt beside me.

'What are you doing?' He nudged his head towards the notepad.

'I'm writing.'

'Do you want to play a game?' he whispered, checking to see if our mums were watching.

'What game?'

'It's a secret. You have to come to my bedroom, but don't let anyone see you, okay?'

'Okay,' I said to his retreating back.

He walked out of the living room and into the darkness of the hallway. I pushed the notepad away and looked into the kitchen, carefully placing the pen on the coffee table. Anisa and Mum were engrossed in their conversation and hadn't seen Fadil talking to me.

My stomach was churning with excitement. Fadil was ten, four years older than me. Like the grown-ups, he overlooked my frowning sallow face and instead focused on my brother's cherubic cheeks and blond curls, but now he actually wanted to play a game with *me.*

With a last look into the kitchen, I stood and stealthily left the living room so Haris didn't see me go. The darkness in the hallway pressed around me. When I reached Fadil's bedroom I knocked softly. Fadil opened the door and pulled me in. The bedroom light was turned off. The streetlight shone through the white blinds, so I could see the outlines of Fadil's bed and student desk.

'The way to play this game is you take off your pants and I take off my pants, okay?' Fadil said, his voice breaking on the last word.

I heard his zipper rasping as he pulled down the tab. He pushed his jeans down his legs, leaving them around his ankles.

'How do you know this game?' I asked, as I pushed my tracksuit pants down my legs, leaving them twisted around my ankles.

'My daddy plays this game with my sister all the time.

Now we take our undies off,' Fadil instructed.

I watched as he pulled his undies down. I could see the outline of his lower body, the pale skinny legs stretching to the floor, but the area between his legs was shadowed. I frowned. It seemed strange and wrong to be showing my pipi to a stranger, but I was emboldened by the darkness and the excitement of receiving Fadil's attention and tugged my panties around my ankles.

A car passed outside, the headlights shining through the blinds and throwing light into the room. For a few seconds the light shone on Fadil. I saw his long thin pipi standing up straight, while his hand tugged on it. The sound of his heavy breathing filled the room as the car engine faded away.

Fadil moved closer and stood over me. His hands pressed against the wall on each side of my head. He bent his knees and started rubbing his pipi between my legs, his breath blowing on my face. He stopped pushing. His body tensed as footsteps sounded down the hallway, heading towards the bedroom. 'Quick, it's my mum,' he whispered. 'Pull up your pants.'

He moved away. I clumsily pulled my tracksuit pants up as the door swung open. Light flooded the room as I released the elastic around my waist. My eyes blinked rapidly as they adjusted to the bright light.

Anisa stood in the doorway, watching us intently. 'Fadil, what are you doing in the dark?' she asked.

'Nothing, Mum.'

Anisa looked at Fadil, the silence stretching between them. 'Go back to the living room and don't come here to play again,' she ordered, her voice harsh. Anisa moved out of the doorway so we could pass.

When we got to the living room I started giggling. 'We'll play the game again when we visit next time,' I said.

He sat on the couch and picked up the remote control. As we watched television I could feel the pressure between my legs, as if Fadil was still pressing his pipi against me.

The next day Mum woke me up, an urgent look on her face. Her eyes were glowing with that strange light that I hadn't yet learnt to recognise. She was in the midst of a euphoric bipolar episode, her eyes shimmering with silver flecks and open wide with surprise and wonder.

'What happened with you and Fadil?' she asked.

'It's a secret,' I said, sleep beginning to clear.

'You can tell me.'

'No, I can't.' I shook my head with emphasis. 'Then it won't be a secret.' I was enjoying the reversal of roles where I had the power.

'Yes, it will. I promise I won't tell anyone,' Mum pleaded.

'Okay,' I finally agreed, eager to share. 'We were playing a new game where you take your pants off and rub your pipis together.'

Mum gasped. 'You can't ever play that game again.' She grabbed my arms and almost shook me. 'Promise me you won't ever play that horrible game again.'

'I promise.' My stomach dropped.

'It's very, very bad to let someone rub your pipi.' There were tears in her eyes and I realised this was not something I should have enjoyed.

I started crying too.

'Good, good,' Mum whispered and left abruptly.

As an adult I realised she must have been terrified and

upset, and had left me so she wouldn't scare me with her crying, but as a child I was left with a scorching shame that coated me from the inside out, tainting me and leaving a residue of rot.

A few weeks later our car broke down and Mum asked Anisa to give us a lift. Anisa's older daughter was in the passenger seat, while Mum, Haris and I sat in the back. I was subdued. Being around Anisa and her family made me uncomfortable. It brought back all the feelings I'd had after talking with Mum.

I was staring out the window and wishing myself away. Mum was agitated and kept shifting around, bumping into me.

'Do you know what game Fadil was playing with Amra?' Mum demanded.

'Kids play,' Anisa said. 'That's what they do.'

'He told her to take off her pants.'

'I'm sure that's not right.'

'He told her to take off her pants and rubbed himself against her,' Mum burst out. 'She told me.'

'Kids make up stories.'

I was angry that Anisa was calling me a liar, but I was angrier with Mum. She'd promised she wouldn't tell anyone and she'd betrayed me. I stared out the window and fantasised about opening the door and throwing myself out of the car. *That would make Mum sorry,* I thought to myself.

Mum was hospitalised again and this time it was my fault: I had played the game and this was the result. A case worker at the hospital asked me and my brother who we wanted to live with, Aida and Zlatan or Hava and Alija. Aida and Zlatan were in the room. I hesitated. I did not want to live with Aida again, with her unyielding, rigid rules, her inability to deal with the natural voice levels of children, but she was right there, listening. Hava and Alija were family; they had lived in the bungalow in our backyard for as long as I could remember.

Haris felt no such qualms. 'Hava and Alija,' he burst out. When the case worker looked at me I nodded. They were familiar and at least I would still be able to go to school.

Later that night, when Hava had made us hot tea and toast before bed, there was a knock on the bungalow door.

'Who is that?' Alija asked suspiciously. Anyone visiting them had to come down the driveway and into the backyard, and it was past the time that polite guests would invade someone's home. He approached the window over the kitchen sink, next to the front door, and lifted the curtain. Standing there were two police officers and a woman with serious faces.

Coldness descended into my bones. The last time the police came they took Mum away. Who were they going to take now?

Alija opened the door.

'Hello, Mr Fehtovic. I'm Lisa, from the Department of Human Services. We've received a notification about children in your care.' She held up a piece of paper with Haris's and my names on it.

'Yes,' Alija said, automatically standing straighter and blocking the doorway.

I hugged Hava and peered out from behind her.

'I'm afraid there have been some concerns raised about their care here,' Lisa said.

'What concerns?'

There was no formal arrangement in place for our care; things were too chaotic. These were family friends offering a hand, not foster carers sanctioned by government bureaucracy.

'That's confidential,' Lisa said. 'I can't divulge that information. We're here to take them into suitable foster care until more permanent arrangements can be made.'

She peered into the bungalow. It was a three-bedroom structure with a detached toilet. The rooms were tiny, the ceilings low, but it was spotless and well-maintained. Like most migrants, Hava and Alija were determined to have their own home, with no mortgage. They lived in the bungalow to save all their money while they built a house a few streets away.

'Amra and Haris are fine with us,' Alija said.

'I'm sorry.' Lisa stepped away from the door and one of the police officers came forward.

'Please move away, sir,' the policeman said. 'Come here.' He gestured to me.

I walked slowly towards the police officer. Haris followed and he was crying, but I felt numb. Alija and Hava walked with us out to the street. We got in the car and the social worker sat in the back with us. I twisted in the seat and watched Alija and Hava through the back window as they got smaller and smaller.

When we turned onto the main street I leaned my head back. I remember seeing the streetlights flash as we drove. We went onto a freeway and I saw the green signs through the back window. We arrived at our destination, and as I was taken into the house I looked at the dark, cold street and fantasised about running away. That was the last thing I remember.

Up until this point we had always been cared for by family friends when Mum was in hospital. Friends of the family, or pseudo relatives. This was the first time we had been put in a stranger's house. The trauma of this experience wiped the slate of my memory clean.

I once spoke to my brother about it and he said that the lady didn't let us play outside – she was probably afraid we'd either try to run away or get lost – and that we mostly ate toast. It would have been traumatic to be without my normal food, my normal friends, or my house. Two days later more suitable arrangements were made and we went to live with Vicky and her family.

I never found out who reported Hava and Alija to the government. Mum suspected that it was their nineteen-year-old son, who was unhappy at losing his privacy in the tiny bungalow. I always wondered if there was more to it than that, and a few years ago I contacted the Department of Human Services to ask for my file under freedom of information. If there was a file, it had been destroyed. The worker told me that it wasn't unusual for files from that generation to have gone missing because record-keeping had been more lax.

Vicky was an approved foster carer. I went to school with Vicky's daughter, Sally, and she took us in while Mum was in hospital. It was my first experience of being with a nuclear family since my father died. I watched, envy twisting inside me, as Sally ran to her father, John, when he came home from work and he caught her in his arms and lifted her up. She searched his pockets to find gum he had bought for her, and when she found her prize she struggled with the wrapping until she could eat it. John would wrestle with his son, Danny, the two of them tussling until they emerged from their scrum rumpled and rosy-cheeked.

A month later Mum was released from hospital and we

were reunited again. We had missed her gentle touch. Vicky served dinner and expected us to eat from the plate without any need of persuasion, while mum always bribed us with a bag of lollies she kept hidden in the kitchen cupboard that we had to earn with our eating.

Mum decided that a visit to Bosnia was in order. She wanted to see her parents, but more importantly she wanted to see my father's grave and lay him properly to rest – in her mind, at least.

MY FATHER'S FOOTSTEPS

The old woman stared at me, awestruck, and cried with her mouth open in raw, uncontrollable sobs. I was terrified and huddled behind my mother's legs. We'd arrived in Bosnia a few weeks before and had set off to visit my paternal grandmother. We travelled on a bus for a day and a night from Bosanska Gradiška, where my mother's family came from, to Travnik, where my father's family lived, chaperoned by my grandfather, who my brother and I called Dido. Travnik, located in central Bosnia, was very hilly; my father came from a village called Gornje Krčevina that was nearly an hour away. We had just arrived in Travnik and were changing buses to go to my father's village when the woman saw me and began crying.

'That's your grandmother.' Dido pushed me towards the crying woman. 'Give her a hug.'

As soon as I was within reach, my grandmother, Kaida, grasped me in a bone-crushing hug. I arched in her arms, trying to get away. She was overcome with emotion at seeing my resemblance to my father. At seven years old I had his colouring: the blue eyes and blonde hair that marked me as different from my mother and her side of the family, who were all dark-haired.

I had inherited my father's high cheekbones and a dimple in the chin that ensured I would hear the phrase 'spitting image' for years to come. This was the first time that someone who saw me after my father's death would have such a strong emotional reaction, but it would not be the last. Over the years many relatives and friends of my father would react with shock at seeing me. Kaida saw my brother (who at this point more closely resembled my mother) and hugged him too.

We travelled with my grandmother by bus to my father's village. The streets got curvier and steeper and there were sections of the road where I looked out the window with awe and fear as the bus seemed to be perched on the edge of a cliff. One wrong turn by the bus driver and we would tumble down to a sure death.

We arrived at the bottom of the hill where there was a *granap*, a Bosnian milk bar. I was tired after being on a bus all day and night, but our journey wasn't done. I didn't know it at the time, but we were about to embark on a lot of climbing.

My grandmother was thin and agile from a lifetime of climbing up and down the hills. We crossed a bridge across the shallow river. I could see white stones on the bottom. The clear water rushing from the mountains made a soothing whooshing noise as it flowed under the bridge.

There were a few houses near the *granap* and beyond them a deep, dark forest. Compared with the bleached tones of Australia's bush the forest looked like a fairytale picture, the greens dark and misty, the brown of the tree trunks like rich, dark earth.

We followed my grandmother across the bridge and began the steep incline. My grandmother led the way, like a leaping goat as her knees bent with the terrain. My grandfather panted at the back, with the compromised chest of a lifelong smoker.

I was able to climb easily, but the pace my grandmother set was too hard for my short legs. My mother was in the middle, helping my brother up while my grandmother forged ahead, not looking back.

We crisscrossed our way up the hills, walking on the edges of fields planted with lush vegetables and bordered by verdant forest. The sound of a cuckoo echoed through the clearing. I recognised the distinctive voice from my grandparent's clock, which sang out every hour in the living room.

We reached the final hill and now had to walk through the forest along a steep path cut into the side by thousands of footprints. I looked to my right where the path ended and felt my stomach drop with fear. One wrong step and I would fall off the trail and roll down, smashing myself on the trees that defied gravity to grow out of the hillside.

My grandmother lived in a little hamlet of ten houses clustered together. Most of them were old-fashioned, built during the Turkish era: the bottom made of wood, the top rendered white, with a red tiled roof. My grandmother's house was new. A double-storey square house with unfinished rooms. Like most Bosnians she built as she saved money. My uncle who worked in Germany sent money, and my father had sent money from Australia. After he died Kaida refunded his return ticket and kept the money.

When we reached the road leading into the village my eyes caught on a cemetery. As I looked around I noticed that each house had a family cemetery beside it. Rather than the dead being hidden away, they were among us, a constant reminder of the preciousness of life. Some of the headstones were hundreds of years old, the concrete pitted and the names faded away.

Goosepimples rose on my skin as I imagined ghosts weaving their way among the headstones and watching me as I passed.

We dropped off our bags at my grandmother's house. I met my cousins, my uncle's daughters, who were being cared for by my grandmother. Sanela was a year younger than me, and her sister was four years old. *Umiđa*, Uncle, had been in a relationship with a Serbian woman and so my cousins were half Bosnian, a fact that I would realise later mattered a lot to my grandmother.

Sanela had been burnt in a house fire and the skin on her legs was twisted and scarred. At first I was fascinated and couldn't look away, but soon enough it became normal. Apparently their mother's lax care was the reason for her burns, and why they were now in my grandmother's care.

My grandmother led us us through the backyard, behind the barn, and to the paddock that was the family cemetery, where my father was buried. Next to him was my paternal grandfather's grave. My mother wept. This was the closure she had been seeking.

My father had returned to Bosnia after he was diagnosed with cancer, planning to say goodbye to his parents and then return home. He was supposed to die in Australia but he stayed too long.

When my grandmother saw my father at the airport she blamed my mum for his emaciated state. 'What has she done to you?' she wailed.

'I'll tell you about my wife,' my father said. 'If she had behaved towards me for six hours the way I did for six years, I wouldn't have stayed for six minutes. Don't ever say anything about her again.'

It had taken a terminal illness for him to acknowledge the pain he had caused, but he never did tell Mum. She heard this story from my grandmother during our visit.

Twenty days after my father arrived, my grandfather had a heart attack and died. Kaida said that my grandfather's heart broke when he saw that his firstborn son was dying. Although my grandfather had been unwell it was believed by all that the stress of his firstborn's diagnosis put his heart under too much strain. My father had extended his stay in order to attend the funeral and to grieve my grandfather's passing with his family. By the time he was ready to use his return ticket, the cancer had other ideas. In Bosnian, *rak* was the word for cancer and for crab, and now my father learnt how the two were intertwined. His body was invaded by these creatures with their vicious claws, and they were eating his body from the inside, ripping apart the sinew, muscle and nerves, leaving him screaming with pain and vomiting blood.

He was admitted to hospital but morphine was scarce, and my grandmother had to purchase it from the black market. I never did learn why. Was it because Yugoslavia, as a communist country, couldn't obtain it? Or perhaps they had to be frugal, and so he was only left with suffering? He had spent his days waiting for my grandmother to appear with the morphine, cursing her for making him come to Bosnia when she returned empty-handed.

Mum told me that she called the hospital. The phone was located in the general office and my father was too weak to walk; instead he was brought in a wheelchair. He told her that he wanted to be with us when he died and vowed that if there was a life after death, he would find a way to be with us again. Mum put me on the phone and I spoke to him for a few minutes before handing back the phone to my mother, telling her, 'Babo is gone.'

Mum heard frantic shouts and movement. After five long minutes a nurse picked up the phone and told her that my father had fallen into a coma. Early in the morning my grandmother called and told her that they expected he would die within the next twenty-four hours. She received the phone call twenty-three hours later.

It was a beautiful summer day when my grandmother took us to the family cemetery behind her house. Mum examined the headstone and collapsed on the grass beside the grave, crying as if it was the first time she had been told about his death. My six-year-old mind was not able to comprehend the sadness of this moment. It wasn't until I visited his grave nearly twenty years later and looked at the years of birth and death that marked his life that I could finally understand the tragedy of his passing. He was only thirty years old.

But in that moment, as my mother wept and my grandmother prayed, I was a carefree child inured from grief. My brother and I played chasey with our cousins in the paddock, the wildflowers and knee-high grass tickling my bare legs as we ran.

When we entered the house again I asked for the toilet. My grandmother had indoor plumbing, but the toilet wasn't connected. Sanela took me to the outhouse behind the barn: a square structure with a door. There was a hole in the floor that I had to crouch over. The excrement rolled down the hill in a kaleidoscope of colour as the different shades of poo mingled together into a fascinating carpet. It was summer and the smell burnt my nostrils.

It took practice to learn to crouch and poo, and it wasn't until my stomach began hurting and my bowels fought to contain all my waste that I learnt to use the facilities, yet even then I spent the whole time with a dreadful fear that I would drop through the hole and into the excrement below, suffocating in the stench.

Dido left after a few days and returned home, while my brother and I remained with Mum. We settled in to village life. There was no school and every day was filled with playing. There were no chores and no expectations. Mum stayed up late and slept in, so I didn't spend much time with her. Seeing my father's grave and learning about his last days had sunk her into a depressive low and she became bedridden and frail – an invisible woman during our stay.

The next day, while Mum was sleeping, Kaida made us breakfast. She had what seemed like a mountain of potatoes and every meal was potato-based. As days passed they got more and more rotten, until she had to cut and throw away more than half of each potato.

I was sitting on the couch in the living room eating potato pita for breakfast.

'Eat, eat,' my grandmother urged.

'I'm full.' I put the plate on the table, while my brother continued eating.

'I'm full too,' Sanela said.

'Eat more,' my grandmother snapped at Sanela.

'I can't.'

Kaika's face changed. She slapped Sanela's bare legs, the

smacking of skin on skin sounding like a gunshot. Sanela wailed from the pain. 'Shut up,' my grandmother shouted. Sanela tried to contain her sounds of pain, but she was still crying. 'I said shut up.' She covered Sanela's mouth and nose with her hand and squeezed her cheeks tightly. My grandmother held her hand there for what seemed like forever. Sanela's eyes showed panic as she couldn't breathe. Finally Kaika removed her hand and Sanela panted shallowly, the sound of a dog choking on a chain.

I sat silently on the couch, too scared to look directly at my grandmother lest she turn her rage on me. But she didn't. My brother and I were the prized grandchildren, the progeny of her favourite son, while my cousins were *Vlahs*, a derogatory term for Christians.

Sanela cried, but quietly. She picked up the plate and ate some more. I did the same. This wasn't the last time I saw my grandmother's brutality towards my cousins. Even though she never laid a hand on me, I feared and hated her.

Grandmother was known for her ferocious temper and cutting tongue. She didn't visit anyone, nor did anyone visit her. Instead, my mother and I made our way around the village by ourselves. When I met the other inhabitants of the village, I realised that we all shared the same surname. It seemed I was related in some way to most of the people who lived there. They were mostly blond with blue eyes so pale I felt like I could see the back of their eyeballs. These were my father's eyes. My eyes were that blue the first year of my life, but then they darkened and became green like my mother's.

There was one woman who fascinated me. Known as the 'mute girl', she lived at the bottom of the hill near the *granap*.

In communist Yugoslavia anyone with a disability was viewed as subhuman, and the deaf-mute woman was shunned in the village. Her disability made her an object of curiosity. Even though she was older than my mum, she had never married and was destined to live out her life caring for her elderly parents. But she was lucky. Most people with disabilities were bundled off to a state-run institution to protect the public from the discomfort of viewing them, letting families hide their shame, but her parents wouldn't allow this.

The first time we met the deaf-mute woman, my mother was startled and couldn't stop looking at her. Dido had returned to take us back to my mother's hometown of Bosanska Gradiška. We were walking down the hill to the bus stop, near the *granap*.

'I need to do one thing,' Mum insisted. She went to the house of the mute girl and hugged her, whispering in her ear. The woman couldn't hear it, of course, so then Mum mimed.

'What did you tell her?' I demanded when we were on the bus. Mum wiped her eyes and shook her head.

I would find out years later what my mother had whispered – and when I did, I would spend a lifetime wishing that I didn't know.

'Leave your mother in peace,' Dido snapped and I quietened down.

I looked out the window at the hills as we passed. We stayed a few more weeks with my mother's parents and then returned to Australia once more.

DADDY SEARCH

One early morning I woke up to find only Haris beside me, so I went searching for Mum. She wasn't in the kitchen or the living room. The door of the spare bedroom was closed. I pushed it open and found Mum naked in bed with a man.

'Mum!' I shrieked. Her eyes opened and she saw me.

Mum had started dating once we returned to Australia a few months before, looking for a husband and father to care for us. Even though she was seen in some circles as damaged goods, she had something that all people desperately dreamt of – her own house, with no mortgage – and this went a long way to making her more desirable. Her dating pool was limited because she only wanted to marry a Bosnian. Being a single mother meant that she was accompanied on dates by my brother and I, or her men had to visit us at home. I was not enamoured with her dating exploits and saw every man as a rival for my mother's affection.

'I'm telling Hava,' I said, knowing that this would be her greatest punishment. Hava would shame her for bringing a man into the house and being so indiscreet that she got caught by her child.

'No,' she gasped.

I started running for the back door. Mum jumped out of bed and chased me. She caught me in the kitchen. 'Please, Amra, please don't tell.'

I met her eyes. She looked scared. I was happy that I had her undivided attention. She sent the man away without letting him linger and made breakfast for us. I had won this round.

Mum's next beau, Muamer, lived in Footscray, a suburb close to the city bordered by the Maribyrnong River. Muamer's house was a white weatherboard with a tin roof and a wraparound porch, in a narrow street built for horse-drawn carriages. After we arrived he led my brother and me back out the front door.

'Over there's a park.' Muamer pointed down the street. 'You two go there and play.'

I sullenly walked to the park. I was seven, old enough to understand why we'd been sent away, but my brother skipped ahead.

When we returned, Mum and Muamer were not in the living room where we'd left them. I ran down the hallway in a panic, Haris following me. Hearing them talking, I pushed the bedroom door open. Muamer was standing beside the bed in a dark blue silk robe that shimmered over his potbelly. The short robe barely grazed his thighs; his hairy legs stuck out the bottom. He looked embarrassed when I walked in. Mum didn't move from where she lay. Muamer picked something up from the bed and headed for the door.

'What's that in your hand?' I demanded, my eyes caught by the stealthy way he crumpled the cloth.

'My socks.' His face turned red. It was his underwear, black cotton briefs.

After he left, Mum looked at us. 'Get out,' she said, her green eyes glowing. As I closed the door I saw her stand up, her pale-fleshed body nude.

Soon, life became unpredictable and strange. Mum had met Muamer on the rebound: she'd thought she'd found the love of her life in her ex-boyfriend, but when we moved in with him and the government threatened to cut off her widow's pension, he cooled on the relationship.

Muamer was not Mum's type or age-appropriate. He had a son that was my mother's age. She never did find out how old he was because he'd scratched out the date of birth on his driver's licence. Mum was twenty-nine and exercised every day to maintain her figure. Muamer was possessive and there were daily fights. Soon he found that he could use his strength to control her.

Muamer's house was old and had no inside toilet; instead there was an outhouse in the small, enclosed concrete backyard. At night my brother and I were too scared to go out. Mum's solution was for us to pee into a bucket that she flushed the next day. Each morning I stared into the bucket, the urine a dark yellow mixture with bits of toilet paper weighing it down, the strong smell wafting up my nostrils.

We were waiting for breakfast while Muamer and Mum shouted. They'd been arguing all morning. Muamer pursued her doggedly around the house, accusing her of flirting with some man or other. Mum tried to go to the kitchen to make breakfast, but he grabbed her by the arms and wrenched her back. 'You are my everything.' His voice was full of pain. I watched from the doorway in my pyjamas as Mum pulled away from him.

'Just tell me you love me,' he pleaded. He grabbed her again but she managed to throw him off. She picked up the pee bucket and tossed it at him. Urine soaked his hair and chest, and bits of toilet paper stuck to his cheeks and shoulder.

'Run.' She yanked us both down the hallway and out the front door.

We ran down the street to the house of a Bosnian family we knew. I kept looking behind us to see if Muamer was following, but he was nowhere to be seen. Mum told the neighbours about the fight, her voice loud as she barely stopped for pause. Her tongue got thick, her speech slurred. The neighbours exchanged looks of concern as they listened to her. They gave Haris and me toast to eat and sent us to the living room to watch television while they remained in the kitchen talking to Mum.

Eventually, there was a knock on the door. The woman of the house answered, leading in Muamer. He looked sheepish, his hair wet.

'He keeps following me,' Mum shrieked. 'He thinks I'm having an affair.'

'Now, now, calm down, Fatima.' Muamer's voice was calm and level. 'There's nothing to be upset about.'

'You never leave me alone,' she shouted. 'I have no peace from you, accusing me of cheating, calling me a slut!'

I snuck to the doorway and saw Mum bunched up against the wall. He was reaching his arms out to her, like she was a wild animal that needed to be contained. The Bosnian couple watched the spectacle.

'Ask Amra.' Mum pointed at me. 'Ask her how he torments me.'

The wife was moved from her inertia – she quickly ran over to me, tugging me away.

'Mummy,' I called out and began crying. 'I want Mummy.'

I tried to push the woman away, but she held onto me as Muamer and her husband led Mum out of the house.

Mum was admitted to hospital. After a few weeks of heavy sedation, Mum stabilised and progressed to weekend visits. On Friday night Muamer would pick her up from the hospital, and on Monday morning he would drive her back.

Haris and I were used to fending for ourselves. With Mum becoming a weekend parent, I settled in to a new life during the week. The playground became my second home and I played there after school until night. I made friends with other neighbourhood children, among them Lucy. Lucy lived a few streets away, but had found her way to our park and it became her daily haunt. She was about my age and we grew close quickly, as children do.

Lucy was always reluctant to go home. I stayed out all afternoon, but when darkness stretched across the playground and Muamer shouted my name from the front porch I didn't linger. While home wasn't a joyful place, it wasn't a place I dreaded. Many nights when I walked towards the shining light on the porch I looked over my shoulder and saw Lucy on the swing, her face etched in sadness as she delayed going home. Muamer didn't allow any kids to visit. My friendships took place in the park and nowhere else.

One weeknight during school holidays, just before Muamer came out to call me home, Lucy asked me if I wanted to sleep over at her house. I'd never had a sleepover at anyone's house before and this seemed like the most exciting thing that could possibly happen. Most importantly, it gave me the chance for a solo experience without my brother.

We ran together to Muamer's house. I yanked open the door and yelled out asking Muamer for permission. I'm not sure why he said yes. Perhaps he didn't understand the concept of a sleepover, or maybe he thought I was asking to visit. It didn't occur to me to pack anything, such as a change of clothes or a toothbrush. We flew off the porch and ran into the darkened streets. Lucy didn't live far away, just a few winding streets down. When we got to her house her mother had visitors so we retreated to her bedroom.

Her house had threadbare carpets and flaking walls. I didn't get the chance to visit many other girls' bedrooms and I was intensely curious. Lucy's bedroom was used as a storage area for her mother's things, and there was barely enough room to walk from the bed to the door. There were clothes on the floor and she didn't have many toys.

The house was quickly filling with adults. Music was turned up loud, and the smell of cigarettes permeated the house. At some point we left the room to eat and entered the crowded living room.

'There's my girl,' her mum drawled. She was holding a beer in one hand and a cigarette in the other. Lucy made her way through the bodies seated on the floor and every available piece of furniture, until we reached the couch where her mother was. Her boyfriend sat beside her. He scooped Lucy up and put her on his lap and tickled her. Lucy didn't look happy, but she didn't get up. After a few minutes enduring the conversation around us, Lucy stood and took me to the kitchen, where we made ourselves a sandwich from stale bread. We returned to her bedroom to eat and then got ready for sleep.

'You have to take off your underwear,' Lucy said, slipping off her panties under the doona and throwing them onto the floor.

'Why?' I asked, finding this strange.

'You just do,' Lucy said and closed her eyes.

Lucy fell fast asleep, untroubled by the shrieking conversation of her mother's drunk and stoned friends fighting to be heard over the throbbing music. I couldn't settle as I lay beside her, with the unfamiliar feeling of bedsheets tickling my private parts, thinking about all the strange things I'd seen and heard. Eventually exhaustion dragged me under.

When we awoke the house was deserted, with remnants of the party strewn all over the living room. Lucy warned me to keep quiet because her mother would be in a bad mood after a hard night. We had a silent breakfast and left the house.

As we walked to central Footscray, Lucy pointed out a house with garden beds neatly planted with colourful rows of plastic tulips. 'Let's get one,' Lucy dared me. I looked back at the house. Something about the way the plastic flowers rose symmetrically out of the garden bed touched my heart. There was beauty in this display and I wondered about the person who had arranged it. Seeing Lucy's wicked smile I realised she didn't share my sentiment and so I nodded. We jumped over the fence and each grabbed a fake tulip and ran away, laughing fiendishly. When we reached the end of the street Lucy threw her plastic flower on the grass. I hesitated before following suit, thinking about the empty space in the flowerbed.

We spent the day window-shopping. At some point we ended up in a toyshop, and envy twisted inside me as I looked at the shelves. I picked up a Cabbage Patch doll and gently caressed her chubby plastic cheek.

'Do you want it?' Lucy asked.

'Yeah, but Mum can't afford it,' I said, regretfully returning it to the shelf. Cabbage Patch dolls were expensive and I'd coveted one ever since I saw the first commercial on television.

'Who said you needed your mum?' Lucy asked scornfully. She looked around us. 'Get ready to run,' she whispered. She grabbed the doll and ran to the door. I hesitated for a split second, shocked at her cunning. My survival instinct kicked in as I realised I was an accessory. We ran until we were again in the quiet suburban streets.

Lucy eventually stopped. I caught up to her and we both bent forward as we fought to get our breath back. 'Here,' she said, a big smile on her face. I took the doll gingerly. I'd dreamt for so long about the moment I finally had my own Cabbage Patch doll, yet now that I finally held one in my arms, it felt tainted.

We spent a few more hours out and about, and when dark approached Lucy asked me again to sleep over at her house.

'I'll have to ask Muamer,' I said cautiously.

'No need,' Lucy said. 'If he said okay once already, he wouldn't have a problem with another night.' This logic seemed to make sense and so I agreed. 'We can't take the doll home, though,' Lucy said.

'Why?' I asked, hugging it tighter.

'Mum will want to know where I got it.'

Something in her face made me not ask questions. I left the doll on a bench, and as dark descended we walked to her house. This time it was quiet with no party; her mum was in the living room, wrapped around her boyfriend. We went to bed, again removing our underwear, and slept.

In the morning my stomach was twisting with hunger. I hadn't eaten much the day before and now I was feeling it. We went to the kitchen, but there was no bread, no milk, no cereal. Lucy's mum came in, her face wan.

'Mum, can you give me money to buy something to eat?' Lucy asked.

Her mum exploded in a rage. 'Shut the fuck up!' She picked Lucy up and threw her against the wall.

My body burst into motion before my mind had time to process it. I ran all the way home to Muamer's house, not looking back once. When I got home, Haris told me that he and Muamer had driven up and down the dark streets of Footscray the night before, searching for me. I expected Muamer to yell at me, but he was too relieved – now he wouldn't have to explain to Mum that he'd lost her child.

WOMAN ON FIRE

The sound of the wind rustling through the trees and a cacophony of birdcalls woke me. My brother was curled against my side inside our shared sleeping bag. Opening my eyes I saw the emerald colour of the nylon tent roof. Through it I could picture the tree branches that we slept beneath twirling in the wind, producing nature's symphony. I lifted my head and saw my mum and Muamer lying on the other side of the tent.

Feeling the press of my bladder I reluctantly unzipped the sleeping bag and slid out, like a critter being born. I pushed open the tent door to a panoramic view of greenery. We had pitched our tent on a clearing surrounded by bushes and trees. As I walked straight ahead to the trees I could hear the river rushing past behind the foliage.

A few metres away there was another tent, for Behija and Eldin and their two sons. Behija was Mum's best friend. Behija and Eldin used to be tobacco sharecrop farmers in Myrtleford and Mum had met them when she lived on a farm with her first husband. They'd invited us on this camping trip, their annual family holiday, to give us the opportunity to reconnect with our half-sister Zehra, Mum's firstborn daughter who lived in Myrtleford with her father.

Muamer wasn't happy that Behija and Eldin had a claim on Mum's affections. He wanted her isolated and vulnerable;

surrounded by friends, she was beginning to show strength.

Our family camping trip was also to celebrate Mum's release from hospital. Mum had been seeing a female Muslim psychiatrist. They had bonded on the basis of their shared religion, and she had triggered a change in Mum.

'What do you think you're doing?' she had demanded when Mum explained that Muamer, a man she barely knew, was caring for her children and that Mum was effectively a weekend parent. 'You keep this up and your children will be taken from you.'

These were the words that slapped her awake. She'd once told me that being in hospital was like a vacation for her. Being a sole parent was a heavy burden for her to carry, but when the psychiatrist made her realise what she was risking, she sought release from hospital and came home.

We spent the days swimming in the lake and bushwalking. Zehra was fourteen years old and spent more time with Eldin and Behija's sons, who were her age, than with my brother and me. She used to visit sporadically, but we'd hardly seen her since our father passed away and our life became tumultuous, and my only memories of Zehra from that time were of her getting us to tidy our room and fold our clothes. I watched with envy as she splashed with the boys, unselfconscious in a white bikini that highlighted her womanly figure.

That night, Eldin and his sons built a fire in the pit they had created away from the tents. We gathered around, the adults sitting on foldaway chairs, while the rest of us sat on logs. Marshmallows, sticks and fire were ready. As we talked, Muamer sipped *rakija*, a Balkan plum brandy, from the bottle he kept at his feet. It didn't take long for the alcohol to fuel his paranoia, and he started making accusations about Mum's chastity.

Muamer couldn't believe that my beautiful mother had chosen him, and he was always on the lookout for betrayal. Her pale, unmarked skin and thin waistline were a stark contrast to his short tubby body, greying hair and the broken capillaries on his nose and cheeks. A smile exchanged with a male acquaintance or an innocent glance at a shopkeeper became events worthy of an inquisition.

'Where were you?' he demanded. 'You were with someone. Who is he?'

Eldin and Behija tried to intervene, but he pushed Eldin away. They retreated, shocked by this violent outburst, probably fearing for their sons' safety. I'm sure they also felt some anger at Mum for putting them in this position; their family holiday was tainted.

Mum tried to move away from Muamer, but he grabbed hold of her, trying to restrain her. They wrestled, moving closer to the fire, when he pushed her. Her arms flailed as she fought to catch her balance. The fire behind her rose bigger and brighter, lighting up her frightened face. A scream trapped in my throat as I watched her fall. She sidestepped in midair, regaining her footing and landing beside the fire pit.

Eldin rushed forward and pushed Muamer back. They argued while Haris and I wrapped ourselves around Mum's shaking thighs. A few minutes later Muamer drove off in a rage, tyres throwing up earth and gravel as he sped off.

He came back the next morning, and we packed up our tent and went home with him. Mum had a lot of time to think on the trip back. Muamer pulled up in the driveway of his house and got out to open the gate, leaving the engine running. While he unlocked the gate, Mum jumped over the gear stick and into the driver's seat. She threw the car in reverse and burst onto the street, the car veering as she sped away from Muamer.

We had nowhere to go, so like a swallow in spring, Mum returned to the only home we'd ever had, the house my father had bought and renovated. A distant female cousin on my father's side was living there with her husband and children. They had just arrived in Australia from Bosnia and were staying in the house while they found their feet.

We pitched our tent under the branches of the mulberry tree I had climbed throughout my childhood. We lay in the tent, the nylon shushing from the wind, as the branches above us rustled. I curled against Mum's side.

'It's my birthday tomorrow,' Mum said with tears in her voice.

'I'll buy you a cake,' I said.

'Thank you, my baby.'

We fell asleep, my brother on one side of Mum and me on the other. My slumber was disturbed by tremors and I forced my eyelids open.

Mum was crying silently, her chest heaving as she held in her sobs. I fell asleep again while the wind witnessed Mum's silent tears. It was her thirtieth birthday.

I woke up Haris and we snuck out before she awoke. We'd slept in our clothes. Mum's purse was on the tent floor. I opened it and took out two gold coins. We walked two blocks to the milk bar, where we picked out a birthday card and a roulade cake. When we got back Mum was still sleeping.

'Happy birthday to you,' we sang softly. Mum sat up in the

sleeping bag, her hair dishevelled, her face creased from the pillow.

'Happy birthday, Mummy.' I handed over the card and the cake. I didn't have a pen and the card was still blank.

'Thank you.' Mum hugged us. Her tears dried in my hair.

After escaping from Muamer we stayed one night in the tent and then Mum took us to a motel that had a swimming pool in the front yard. My brother and I had our bathers from the camping trip. Mum supervised us splashing and playing in the water while lying on a stripey banana lounge chair, wearing jeans and a pink top with three-quarter sleeves.

She stood and walked to the edge, staring at the water for a moment. Suddenly she jumped in and I watched her sink to the bottom. My heart raced as I waited for her to come to the surface. She swam the length of the pool and got out, lying back down on the banana lounge, fully clothed and dripping wet.

'Mum, why didn't you get your bathers?' I asked.

Mum didn't answer. She closed her eyes and sunbathed. Vapour rose from her clothes as she dried. I was perturbed but I continued playing with my brother.

We remained at the motel for a week, until we got our furniture back from Muamer and moved into the bungalow behind our house. Alija and Hava had moved out after they finished building their house, and their son had left behind his fish tank. Haris and I cleaned it and badgered Mum into buying fish. I was so proud walking out of the pet shop carrying my plastic bag. We put them into the fish tank and found them dead the next day. A schoolfriend explained that fish need a filter for their water and that's why they died.

Mum wanted to flush the fish down the toilet, but I

refused. I'd watched a movie where baby alligators that had been flushed grew in the sewers, eating unsuspecting humans who had to work there. We buried our fish in the backyard. I wanted to get another fish and a filter, but Mum refused.

Mum enrolled us in a school. She made us lunch every day and walked us to school and waited for us at the gate when we finished. As we walked back we'd pass by a park and she'd sit on a bench and watch us play while having a conversation with one of the other mums. We were just regular school children, with a regular mum.

Our small oasis ended much too soon. Muamer started following us: whenever Mum drove, Haris and I saw him through the back window. Soon his daily stalking wasn't enough and he became bolder. I was in a deep sleep when his droning voice intruded. I opened my eyes and saw Muamer outside our bedroom window. He'd brought a folding chair and a bottle of *rakija*.

'Why did you leave me, Fatima?' he demanded plaintively. 'I loved you so much. Took care of you. Took care of your children.' He took a sip from the bottle. 'You are so ungrateful. You don't appreciate all the sacrifices I made for you.'

'Mummy, make him go away,' Haris said, crying.

As Mum covered his ears and pulled him against her I saw the helplessness on her face.

This became Muamer's nightly ritual. He'd spend hours sitting on the chair, sipping *rakija*, as rants spilled from his lips. He'd rave on about how much he loved Mum and wanted her to be with him, begging her to take him back. Interspersed with his supposed declarations of love were rants about Mum's betrayal in leaving him.

There was only one bedroom and we had nowhere else to sleep. I'd have trouble falling asleep listening to his rants, but eventually exhaustion would take hold and drag me under. His droning voice became background noise, until his intonation changed and his voice got louder. Then I'd wake up and glance over at his angry red face, but eventually fall asleep again.

When I couldn't sleep I fantasised about sneaking through the bungalow, carefully opening the front door so he didn't hear, and creeping around the corner with an axe. I would catch him by surprise, raising the axe above my head and striking a blow to his head. While he lay splayed on the ground I would keep striking, hacking him to pieces.

Worn out by his stalking, Mum decided that the only way we could escape him was to leave the country. She booked our tickets to Bosnia, hoping that we would be taken care of by her parents and extended family and it would give her the opportunity to recover.

Up until now all our moving had been dictated by Mum's hospital admissions. This time I was eight years old and it was the first time that I could prepare to leave. I had settled in at school and every lunchbreak was a chance to play. As the time approached for us to go, I began to feel a sense of loss – I'd said goodbye to friends, schools, homes, so many times, but usually I was yanked out of my routine and my life. This time I knew it was coming; I could take it on board, process it, feel sadness about leaving and excitement about going on holiday.

I didn't realise it at that time but I was prescient in saying goodbye: I would never again be a primary school student in Australia. I was about to embark on a new phase of my life and nothing would ever be the same.

PART II

ARRIVAL

I stared at the floor as I danced from foot to foot, the pressure of my full bladder building. We were on our way from Belgrade airport to my grandparents' house and this was our first toilet stop. The only problem was this was unlike any toilet I'd ever seen. There was a hole in the ground with a metal platform around it. As I squatted and the stream of urine went into the hole, I felt my waning excitement sputter and die at the thought of having to use toilets like this.

My mother's sister Nermina – who I called Tetka, which means 'maternal auntie' in Bosnian – and her husband, Damir, had picked us up from the airport. I stared out the window as Damir (who was Tetak to me) drove. I was struck by the greenery. The landscape was unlike anything I'd seen in Australia. The greens were brilliant, and it looked like giant Christmas trees lined the streets. Even the light was different. Australia's sun was like a voltage lamp turned up high so that it leached all the colour out of the landscape, while Europe with its diffused light was like a dim lamp.

It was a four-hour drive to get to my grandparents' house in Bosanska Gradiška. The town was on the right bank of the Sava River, which marked the border between Bosnia and Croatia. The Balkan War treaty made the town a part of Serbia in 1992, but in the summer of 1985 when I arrived as an eight-year-old, Bosanska Gradiška belonged to Bosnia and Hercegovina.

When my mother left home she was fifteen years old and my grandparents lived in a two-bedroom house with no inside plumbing. They had bought a large tract of land that used to be flooded before the canal was dug and then promptly had to sell off parcels before the Communist government confiscated it. This, coupled with my grandfather's new-found religious fervour, had ensured their prosperity.

My grandfather had extended the original abode into a four-room house with a separate kitchen and an indoor bathroom. They were almost completely self-sufficient. They had a one-hectare plot with a fruit orchard at the front with cherries, black and white grapes, and apples, and grew a vegetable harvest at the back. There was also a barn with two cows, whose milk provided all of their dairy products, a chicken coop, and a shed where my grandfather had a flour mill. Villagers from all around came to him with grain and corn, which he would grind into flour for a fee. They also owned acres of land in various other villages that they used to harvest hay to feed the cows.

A full house greeted us. I didn't remember much about the trip we'd made after my father died, and I didn't recognise all the family who were now waiting for me. There were my three cousins, Tetka and Tetak's children, my maternal uncle Reif (who I called Dajđa) and his wife, Dinca, and of course my grandfather, Dido, and my grandmother, Nana. There was a lot of crying and hugging and touching and talking. There was an outpouring of emotion, but there was only one thing I was interested in. I went to the bathroom as soon as I had a chance and breathed a sigh of relief when I saw the upright toilet.

Nana showed me to the bedroom that I would share with Mum and Haris. There was no bed, only a fold-out couch. In fact, there were no beds in the whole house: all the couches folded out. When I visited other houses I discovered that not many people had beds, and most of them slept on fold-out couches to conserve space – the living room by day becoming a bedroom at night.

Because Mum had decided that this was going to be an extended stay, she had enrolled me in school. We arrived during the school holidays, which meant that first I got to enjoy a golden summer. At six years old Haris was too young: children there began school at seven, so he got one more year of freedom.

The village children played outside late into the night. An empty paddock a few houses away was our base. We played everything and anything: chasey, hide-and-seek, ball games.

One night I ran into the house, my stomach aching from hunger. Nana cut me a slice of *pogača*, homemade bread, and slathered a thick layer of jam on it. I left the house, eating the bread on the run. When I finished the slice I felt hungry again. All the running around had opened up my appetite. I returned to the house another four times.

'Are you eating it all yourself?' Dido demanded, looking at me with suspicion.

'Yes, I am.'

'She must be sharing it with the other kids,' Dido said.

'No, I'm not.' I was angry that he didn't believe me.

'You have to eat inside,' Dido said.

Nana served me my slice of bread at the kitchen table. Sitting down to eat meant that the food actually stuck to my stomach and I finally felt full.

'Do you want any more?' Dido asked. I shook my head. 'Like I said, she was sharing food with the other children.' Dido smiled, happy he'd been proven right. I left to play again, not understanding why it was so bad for me to share food and why my grandfather didn't believe me.

That was our last summer of freedom. The main road in front of my grandparents' house was unsealed, so any cars that did come through would drive slowly as they bounced over the potholes. By the next summer the road had been asphalted and it became a busy thoroughfare, with cars and trucks thundering in both directions. A few weeks after the road was finished, my Tetka was buying ice-cream for her children from a ice-cream truck across from her house. Her five-year-old son grabbed his ice-cream and went to run across the road, something he had done hundreds of times before. A car hit him, dragging him underneath it for 45 metres as the driver desperately braked, leaving black skid marks. My cousin survived, but our innocence was gone. The village children never played near the road again.

Winter was a revelation. It brought snow, sub-zero temperatures and the dreaded flu that I contracted each and every New Year's Eve that necessitated home remedies such as cut potatoes in socks or socks drenched in homemade *rakija* to stop the fever.

But winter also meant a magical time of play. There was pretend skating in our worn-down rubber boots on the canal behind my grandparents' house. As Bosanksa Gradiška was flat and I didn't have a sleigh, my experience of sledding was the slope of the canal and a plastic bag. It was magic to fly down the slope at speed and then slide across the bottom of the canal until I finally stopped. At least, it was until the snow thinned and protruding rocks jolted painfully into my tailbone.

While I loved being able to enjoy carefree childhood games, being a child again came at a price. My grandparents were old-fashioned and believed children's innocence should be protected. I was watching television with my grandparents when the lead characters began kissing. Dido turned to me and Haris. 'Go outside.' He pointed to the living room door, which led out to the draughty hallway.

I looked at him in surprise. 'Why?'

'Because these are things children should not see,' Dido said.

'They're just kissing.' I pointed to the TV screen, but things had progressed and now the male actor had his hand on the woman's breast. I had watched many movies with Mum where the man and woman did more than kissing.

'Out now!' Dido shouted.

I looked at Mum, but she didn't look at me. Haris and I went out into the hallway, where we could still hear the sounds of lovemaking. A few minutes later the door opened; Nana could reach the doorknob from the couch. We came back in and continued watching.

A few days later the vet arrived and I followed my grandparents to the barn. I didn't know it at the time, but he was there to artificially inseminate the cow. I frowned as the vet pulled on plastic gloves that reached his shoulder, trying to figure out what was going on.

'I need someone to hold the cow.' The vet bent over his case.

'I'll do it,' I said from the doorway. No one reacted. I was nonplussed. Had I imagined I was speaking? 'I'll do it,' I said again. Again no one answered. Embarrassment descended as I realised that it wasn't that they hadn't heard me – they were wilfully ignoring me.

Dido gave me a look, the look that said I needed to make myself scarce. I retreated into the yard, angling myself so I could still see through the doorway without them noticing.

The vet moved to the back of the cow and lifted her tail. He pushed his hand in; it took me a moment to understand that he was pushing his hand inside the rectum in order to reach the cervix. He scooped the faeces out and wiped the entrance. He then pushed his hand back inside, holding the rod that contained the semen. As his hand disappeared to the elbow I finally knew why he was wearing such long gloves.

Later I asked Mum, 'Why did they pretend I wasn't speaking?'

'Because you're a young girl. You're not supposed to know about these things.'

'What things? Like where a pipi goes?'

'Yes.' Mum looked around uneasily. 'Young girls aren't supposed to know those things. A young girl is supposed to be protected.'

'Is that why they send me and Haris out of the room whenever there is a love scene?'

'Yes.'

'But that's stupid.'

Mum shrugged. 'That's the way things are here. We're living

with your grandparents now and we have to follow their rules.'

A year later, when I began watching television in secret with my grandmother, I got to watch one of the love scenes my grandfather had been protecting me from. The man placed a tea towel over the woman's face and then climbed on top of her. As I watched I wasn't shocked – I already knew more than the other children I played with. Instead, I was curious about why he'd covered her face and, more importantly, why she let him do it.

TRUE BELIEVER

My grandfather was a man of contradictions. I once found him huddled behind the logs waiting to be sawed for winter firewood, weeping because my grandmother had trapped and killed a snake that had been hunting our chicks. Yet he was also capable of great rage and violence. He once threw a handsaw at my grandmother, striking her on the torso. Thankfully the sharp saw teeth were turned away, leaving mottled bruises instead of broken skin.

It was this ability to live between extreme emotions that imbued his stories with heartfelt reality during the four years I lived with my grandparents in Bosnia.

My grandparents greeted each morning with a pot of thick Bosnian coffee. As my brother and I ate our breakfast we would listen to our grandfather's stories. Dido sat on the wide couch that doubled as my grandmother's bed, with his feet off the floor so that his knees were against his chest. He took up hardly any space. He was a short man with a slim build. The family joke was that he was built like a prepubescent boy because the rage that fuelled him was like a furnace burning his body fat. His bed was the narrow couch on the other side of the room that he folded out every night.

Nana hobbled as she brought out the tray with two eggs, coffee and *fildžani* – demitasse coffee cups. Rheumatoid arthritis had eaten away at the cartilage between her knee joints, making the bones rub against each other and causing pain to shoot through her legs with each step.

She'd been slim in her younger days, but over the years the Bosnian fare of starchy bread, oily food and sweets, combined with her rheumatism, meant that she'd reached 100 kilos long ago. When she sat the couch it dipped slightly, and she had to push the tray closer to my grandfather so it didn't topple over.

As Nana poured, the thick coffee glistened in the bright morning sun. Dido picked up an egg and a skewer. He skilfully made a small hole at one end of the egg and then made a larger one at the other end. He placed his lips on the large hole and sucked out the raw egg, swallowing it in one gulp.

He'd been drinking two raw eggs every morning since his heart attack a year before – a home remedy he insisted would stave off another attack. After he'd drunk both eggs he left the empty eggshells on the tray and lifted a *fildžan*, cupping it in both hands.

'Every child is born with its destiny written on its forehead,' he said, as he took his first sip. His mouth looked like a cavernous clown mouth, his gums gleaming pink.

Like a lot of people in the village, he'd lost most of his teeth from decay at an early age. He'd had full dentures made but he never wore them, and so his face had sunk into itself, making him look like a walking skull. His modified diet, which pandered to his tender gums, was probably responsible for his thin build.

My brother and I sat at the kitchen table opposite my grandparents, sipping homemade rosehip tea and eating a thick slice of Nana's *pogača* coated in sour cream. I watched Dido and waited for him to continue his story.

'There once was a woman who birthed a baby girl,' Dido said. 'The woman was very poor and she cursed her fate that she had a child she could not provide for.'

He slurped another sip of coffee, while I swallowed the *pogača* that had been sitting in my mouth.

'She was going to be a prostitute,' Nana said.

'*Zaveži Stara*,' Dido snapped, telling the old woman to shut up. He did not appreciate anyone interfering during his sermons.

The ticking of the cuckoo clock on the wall above my grandparents was the only sound in the room. Nana poured again. Even though she physically dwarfed my grandfather, she had learnt to remain silent when he spoke.

'It was written on the baby's forehead that she would provide for her mother by being a prostitute,' Dido continued. 'The mother was determined that she would not meet this fate and be shamed by her daughter, so she slit the baby's throat.' Dramatically, he demonstrated a slashing motion with his hand.

I blinked, horrified and riveted.

'The child was buried in the cemetery and her mother visited her grave every day. Unknown to the woman, some coffee beans had been mixed with the earth of her daughter's grave and a coffee plant grew. The woman harvested the coffee beans and was able to trade them for food, and thus her daughter's fate came to pass and she provided for her mother.'

After Dido finished I had so many questions. Did the woman regret killing her child? Wasn't she put in jail? But I swallowed my questions the way I did the *pogača*.

My grandfather did not encourage questioning minds.

He told his stories to educate us about Islam and to inspire us to believe. A fervent communist in his youth, he had found faith in his mature years. He saw it as his duty to indoctrinate his Australian grandchildren, and thus we were subjected to his daily religious stories disguised as parables.

He told us stories about being a soldier during World War II. When we asked if he killed anyone, he looked forlorn. 'I closed my eyes as I pulled the trigger,' he'd tell us. He never ate cucumber and even the smell made him retch. He told us about his father, who used to beat his family and they would have to hide out in the cornfield until his rage abated. Dido had never been fond of cucumber. One night he refused it and his father beat him, forcing him to eat it, even after he vomited again and again.

My favourite stories were the ones my grandfather told about how he discovered his faith. In their youth my grandparents travelled around Yugoslavia as migrant workers. Their circumstances were sometimes desperate as they moved between substandard housing and backbreaking jobs. My grandfather was an alcoholic and what meagre income they earned would sometimes be squandered at the bar when he shouted all the men drinks. There were days when there wasn't enough food. On one such day he ran from the house, tormented by the cries of hunger from his two daughters, then an infant and a toddler.

It was winter and snowing. He found himself on a bridge above a river, looking down at the ice floating by. His despair and self-loathing congealed into a need for escape. He leapt off the bridge with his eyes closed, wanting to take his pain away. He landed on a large sheet of ice and automatically clutched at it, his legs immersed in the freezing water. Before he could gather himself, the ice was propelled to shore by the river current.

When he arrived home and told my grandmother what had happened, she was outraged. 'Promise you won't do that again,' she begged as she helped him take off his wet clothes. As she wrapped him in a blanket and watched him shiver, a shudder of fear passed through her. While my grandfather's alcoholism made life hard for him and his family, life without a husband almost guaranteed death by starvation for her and her children.

My grandfather attempted suicide another two times. He tied a rope to a beam in the shed where he worked, climbed on a tractor and jumped. The rope broke and he landed on the ground, knocking himself unconscious. He awoke with a burn mark around his neck and a bump on his head as mementos.

The final time was when my mother was a child. She saw him walking into the woods with a rope and knew what he was planning. She got my grandmother, who collected an axe and ran after him. They found him hanging from a tree, his legs kicking, his tongue protruding as he began the dead man's dance.

My grandmother climbed up and chopped him down. He landed on the ground and spasmed for a moment, before leaping to his feet and running. It took three men a kilometre to catch him and bring him back, teary and shivering with shock.

After his third failed suicide attempt, he decided that this was a sign that God had plans for him. A sign that he had to change his life. A sign that God didn't want him yet. So he turned his attention to making his life a worthwhile endeavour and embraced Islam, his true-born religion.

My grandfather told me that our ancestors were Bogumils. When translated, Bogomil means 'dear to God', as it is a compound of the Slavic words for 'God' (*bog*) and 'dear' (*mil*). The Bogumil sect, which rejected Christianity, was founded in Bulgaria in the tenth century. The Bogomils eventually created a Bosnian Church and were considered heretics by the Catholic and Orthodox churches. It is believed that after the Ottoman Empire invaded they converted to Islam.

My grandfather was raised in a religious household. He moved away from his faith when he became a member of the Communist Party in his youth, only to return in middle age. He adhered to the tenets of his religion: he began praying five times a day and following the five pillars of Islam. But it was his lifelong addiction to alcohol that would present his greatest trial and test of faith.

The first time my grandfather vowed to stop drinking was after the birth of his first grandchild. As he held her in his arms and cupped her head with his hand he swore he would not drink another drop. Within months he broke that promise. The second time, he walked to the cemetery and stood at his mother's grave and made the vow. But the devil tempted him again. The third and final time he held a Qur'an in his hand and swore to God as a witness that he would not drink again. Allah heard his vow and the devil lost his hold, and so a believer was born on that day.

Even though I found Dido's stories disturbing, I loved being the centre of his attention for those few minutes. A man typical of his generation, my grandfather never had much time for the women in his life. It was my brother who got to accompany him on his trips around the village, hanging onto the tractor like a mascot as Dido drove, while I remained behind with my grandmother. But in these quiet moments, when my brother and I were the only audience available, my grandfather spoke to me.

'Allah knows best,' Nana said.

'That's right,' Dido agreed, giving her a dirty look for interrupting. 'Allah in all his glorious knowledge knows what is best for each of us and our destiny is written before we are born and we can do nothing to escape it.'

My grandmother's stories were very different from my grandfather's. She was illiterate and through her sixty years of marriage she had learnt to lose herself in her imagination. She had a childlike love of movies and stories and we spent many an hour watching television together and discussing the characters as if they were our friends.

After my grandparents drank their coffee, Dido would leave the house to run errands or work outside with Haris, and this was my time alone with Nana. Nana rolled up her *dimije* and lay on the couch. I poured cream on my hands and commenced massaging her sore legs.

The burden of housework and farm work fell to my grandmother, exacerbating her rheumatism. Her day began when she woke up at five o'clock, well before dawn lit up the sky. The cuckoo clock on the living room wall sung all day and night on the hour, and my grandmother's internal alarm clock was primed to recognise when it sang out five times.

While we all slept, she sat up on the couch and put on her

dimije (which are similar to harem pants with a drawstring waist tie, and are only worn by peasant women in villages) and put a blouse on over her nightie. Her waist-length salt-and-pepper hair was tied in a long plait that started out thick at top and became a thin cue at the tip. She wrapped her plait around her hand and held it on top of her head as she tied a šamija around her head, trapping the plait within the fold of the headscarf. She folded her bedding and then quietly walked to the small kitchen attached to the living room where she and Dido slept, and stoked the fire in the stove before leaving the house.

She hobbled to the garage that housed the tractor and there donned her milking clothes: black knee-high boots and a blue work smock. My grandmother's first job was cleaning up manure and feeding hay to the cows, then she filled a metal bucket with water and washed the cows' teats. Sometimes she had to wash the manure off a cow's tail if it had caked dry; otherwise, if the cow swished its tail to dislodge flies, it could hit her in the face like a whip. She put a fresh bucket under the cow's teats and sat on her small wooden stool. After she finished the milking she poured the fresh milk into the metal milk bucket, with a piece of muslin cloth on top to strain it, and sealed the lid so it didn't get contaminated.

When both cows had been milked she changed out of her milking clothes and hung them up to air. She carried the milk bucket and left it on the front stairs, then went out to the chicken coop to collect the freshly laid eggs and feed the chickens grain. Afterwards, she carried the eggs and milk back to the house.

While Nana boiled milk for coffee and water for tea for me and Haris, Dido woke up and performed his ablutions before praying. He'd bring a tin cup of boiling water, his shaving cream and a straight-backed razor to the couch. First he'd comb his hair, using the comb that he always kept in his back pocket, and then he'd slick it back with hair cream. He had a receding hairline, but what hair he had left was thick and black.

Next he'd slather his face with shaving cream, carefully using the razor to shave until his skin was smooth. Finally came the aftershave. By the time he returned to the living room, Haris and I were awake and observing his morning rituals, while Nana prepared the morning coffee and our breakfast.

Once my grandfather left for the day, she had a short respite before she had to bake bread, cook a meal, and then begin the afternoon cleaning of the barn and milking of the cows.

'Nana, tell me a story,' I begged as I massaged her legs, the methylated cream filling my nose and making my hands tingle.

'Once there was a slothful housewife,' my grandmother began, her voice drowsy as she relaxed while I kneaded her flesh. 'She didn't clean her floors or wash her dishes properly, and no one ever visited her. This woman was so lazy that she never folded her clothes – instead she threw them in the wardrobe and plucked out what she would wear. Everyone knows that this is the way to invite the devil into your house,' my grandmother warned.

'One night someone woke her calling her name. When she went outside there was a huge bonfire and beside it was a man roasting a cob of corn. He was handsome and well-dressed, and he offered her some to eat. As the slothful housewife lifted the corn to her lips a woman's voice called her name. It was a *villa*, warning her not to eat.' In most of my grandmother's stories there was a *villa*, the Bosnian name for a fairy that issued warnings and helped people. 'The woman dropped the corn and it fell onto her nightgown. The man and the bonfire disappeared. She woke up the next morning marvelling at this strange dream. As she got out of bed she noticed corn smeared on her nightgown.'

For years after hearing her story I folded my clothes neatly, terrified of calling the devil to tempt me. My grandmother's stories were always about fairies and devils. Stories full of magic and wonder. Stories that inspired belief in things we could not see or hear. Looking back I think she needed to believe in a world beyond the one we can see in order to cope with the life she was trapped in.

I only asked my grandmother once how she came to marry my grandfather. Her face became closed off and she sat up, cutting her massage short. It was ten years later when my mother told me their story and I finally understood my grandmother.

After World War II, when my grandmother was sixteen years old, a woman without her virginity intact would bring shame on her family and have no prospect of marriage. My grandmother's brothers were able to come and go as they pleased, but she and her sisters always missed out.

When my grandmother and her sister Lamia overheard that their older brother Enes was going to a party, they blackmailed him into letting them go with him. Enes tried to tell them it wasn't the kind of party women attended, but they wouldn't listen.

When they arrived they found that the party was actually an excuse for Enes and his friends to drink *rakija* and play cards. My grandmother wanted to leave, but Lamia convinced her to stay.

When they were offered *rakija*, Lamia took a sip and waved a hand in front of her mouth. 'Try it, Adevija,' she encouraged my grandmother, taking another big gulp.

My grandmother took a sip. Her face scrunched up as it dried her mouth, her eyes burnt and she nearly choked. Everyone laughed, including Lamia. As the hours passed my grandmother sat stiffly, holding the full glass and pretending to sip every few minutes. She didn't want them to laugh at her again.

My grandmother noticed Enes leaving, but she assumed he was going to the latrine. She couldn't have imagined that his anger would extend so far as to leave them alone and unchaperoned. When an hour passed and he didn't return she understood the truth, but it was too late.

Unaccustomed to alcohol, Lamia had passed out, and my grandmother found herself alone with my grandfather and his friend. She noticed the way they were looking at her and she soon realised that their intentions were less than honourable, but she couldn't leave her sister behind.

Finally my grandfather's friend propositioned her. 'You can choose one of us to marry or we will both have you,' he said.

She fought for breath as panic filled her, her eyes dancing between the two men. She realised her fate had been sealed the moment she decided to stay at the party.

She lifted her arm and pointed.

SPARE THE ROD

My mother sat on a kitchen chair holding a wooden rod. She patted her thighs, indicating I should lie down bare-arsed across her lap to receive my punishment. My heart sped up and my muscles tightened, ready to launch me into a run out the front door, but the realistic part of me began walking slowly towards my mother. After all, even if I ran away, I would have to return at some point.

It had all begun a few months before when my mother and Dido attended parent–teacher interviews.

'Your daughter is experiencing some issues,' my teacher told them. 'While she has acclimatised to the language, she hasn't been completing her homework.'

'We'll make sure it doesn't happen again.' Dido gave me a dark look from under his eyebrows, while Mum nodded wordlessly.

I was eight years old when we arrived in Bosnia and I was placed in the second grade. Mum bought all the necessary supplies to equip me for school, but it was my grandmother who took over the school routine. School in Bosnia was divided into alternating morning and afternoon shifts: morning shift began at eight and ended at midday, while the afternoon shift began at one and finished at five. When I attended morning shift my grandmother woke me, and Mum went outside and completed the chores while Nana fed me before I walked to school.

School in Bosnia was very different to the Australian approach to education. I struggled with the Yugoslavian system, which was focused on rote learning with no opportunity for individual opinion or creative expression.

When Mum returned home from parent teacher interviews my grandparents told her that my efforts were not acceptable. Academic failure brought embarrassment and shame, and while no one in our extended family had a university qualification (in fact, my grandparents hadn't completed high school), this was seen as yet another example of my mother's parental failure.

'You need to show her who is boss. She has no respect for you,' Nana said. 'It's as if you're not her mother.'

My grandmother had struck a nerve. Mum felt that she was lacking as a parent, after all those times when she wasn't able to take care of me and Haris and strangers had to step in. Now it was time for her to take charge and ensure my academic success. The first step was forcing me to comply with homework.

I was sitting at the kitchen table reciting the multiplication times tables while Mum and Nana prepared lunch. Dido had taken Haris out with him to run errands while the women remained at home and did the real work. It was a beautiful summer day and the window was open, letting in the calls of children playing outside.

'Mum, I want to go outside to play.'

Mum opened her mouth to answer, but Nana jumped in before she could say anything. 'She can't go out to play. She has to study.'

'Have you learnt your times table?' Mum asked.

'Yes.' I sat up straighter.

'Test her,' Nana urged.

Mum picked up the textbook. 'What is two times two?'

'Four.'

By the time Mum got to six times six I was flagging and making errors. 'You need to study more.' Mum returned the textbook to the table.

I tried to study, but my concentration was shot. I kept sighing and wiggling in my seat, stretching my arms and legs. Each time I heard a child's shriek or peal of laughter my head bobbed up and I looked out the window. 'Mum,' I pleaded. 'Please, I've learnt it all.'

Mum hesitated. I knew she wanted to let me have a break – I had been studying for an hour and a half – but when she turned to look at Nana, she shook her head and Mum answered, 'No.'

'Mum, please,' I pleaded again fifteen minutes later, on the verge of tears.

Nana leaned forward and whispered in Mum's ear. 'Okay, you can go if you think you have learnt the times table, but I'm going to quiz you later and for every answer you get wrong I will spank you,' Mum said.

As I ran out to the street to play, I felt a qualm. My mother did not make idle threats. She had implemented a warning system for Haris and my misbehaviour, and the third time we misbehaved we got a spanking. There was only one time that Mum hadn't followed through, and my brother and I delighted in reminding her months later. I was six years old and my brother four. We'd been on the road after visiting family friends who lived over an hour away. We'd got bored and begun playing and screaming in the back seat, making Mum too anxious and stressed to concentrate on driving.

Mum had given us three warnings and we finally quietened down, falling asleep before we got home. Mum had carried us to bed. By the time morning came around she'd forgotten all about following through with the spanking, and it was months before we gleefully reminded her about it.

I knew that when I returned, Mum would spank me if I failed the test, but I thought a wooden spoon on the bottom was a small price to pay for a few hours of bliss.

While I was gone Nana left the house and returned with a *motika*, a thin branch that she had plucked all the leaves from.

'What's this for?' Mum asked as my grandmother handed it to her.

'For Amra.'

'No, I use a wooden spoon.' Mum tried to return the *motika*.

'Well, obviously that's not working, so you need to try something new. You need to use this and teach her a lesson.'

Mum's stomach cramped with anxiety. She'd never enjoyed spanking us, and every time she had to do it her whole body seized with dread. Having been on the receiving end of beatings, Mum abhorred violence and only used corporal punishment because she needed something to scare us into submission. Mum wanted to refuse the *motika* and throw it away, but she was living on my grandparents' mercy.

When I returned Mum lifted the textbook and quizzed me on the times tables. I made seven mistakes. My grandmother was sitting on the sofa. She bent over to pick up the *motika* from the floor and handed it to Mum.

I looked at Mum with fear and confusion. Mum pulled a kitchen chair out from under the table and sat down. 'Come here, Amra.' She patted her thighs.

I approached slowly.

'Drop your pants,' Nana said from behind us.

Mum didn't look at my grandmother. She wanted this over and done with. She quickly yanked me towards her and pulled my pants down, baring my buttocks, as she pushed me down across her lap. The *motika* made a whizzing sound as she lifted her hand and then a there was a sharp crack as it hit my bare skin. I flinched in her lap and screamed as Mum delivered the seven blows.

When Mum finished I stood and pulled my pants up.

'There, now she knows not to shirk her study,' Nana said as I ran out of the room.

Later that night Mum ran the bath water and waited for me and Haris to get in. I sullenly took off my clothes, pulling off my pants and revealing the red welts cutting across the skin of my buttocks. I gently rubbed my fingers across the welted flesh and looked at Mum. Mum shrunk at the hatred in my eyes. She told me that in that moment I looked just like my father and Mum felt like she was seeing a ghost. Then the moment passed and once again she saw me as an eight-year-old, so skinny that she could count my ribs.

I turned away and got in the bathtub, wincing as the hot water burnt my skin. Mum was overwhelmed with guilt. After growing up with my grandfather using his fists indiscriminately, Mum had promised herself that she would never strike her children in anger, and she'd kept her promise by always using a wooden spoon. Even when she was frustrated by our behaviour, in the time it took her to find a wooden spoon and mete out her punishment, she had a chance to calm down and make sure she did so sparingly.

But this was different. She had never used a *motika*, and she had never been so harsh before. 'I'm sorry,' Mum said as she wrapped a towel around me after my bath. I resisted for a moment before resting my head on Mum's shoulder.

After that day both Mum and I learnt our lesson: it was my grandmother who was the parent and we were both her children.

HOMECOMING

My grandmother sent me to answer the front door. On the doorstep I found a woman I'd never seen before, holding my mother by the arm. 'Can you get your nana or dido?'

My mother was looking around with glassy eyes and a vague face. 'I want to go shopping,' she slurred, sounding as if she was drunk.

'It's okay. You'll go shopping later.' The woman patted my mother's arm as she placated her.

I returned and Nana followed me, frowning because she hated being interrupted. The woman was a customer of Dido's flour mill. She had found my mother in town, she told Nana in a hushed whisper, even though no one else was around. Some mercenary acquaintance had been leading her through the *Robna Kuća*, the only department store in our town, and picking out expensive household goods for Mum to purchase.

'I told them they were being unethical, taking advantage when it's obvious she is not well. I took what she bought them.' She handed Nana a plastic bag. Nana peered inside to find a crystal vase and glasses. 'But I think she'd been in town for a while and has probably spent a lot of money.'

'Thank you very much. Come inside for coffee?' Nana asked her.

'No, I can't impose. I will come by another time.' The woman walked away briskly.

Nana held the door open. 'Come inside now, Fatima,' she told my mother curtly.

'What were you thinking?' Dido shouted.

'You have embarrassed us in front of all our neighbours,' Nana said.

While my grandparents had heard about my mother's nervous breakdowns in Australia, this was the first time they had been confronted with the reality. They believed that all they had to do was 'talk sense' into my mother; they didn't understand that her illness was beyond her control and theirs.

My mother had brought a supply of her medication to Bosnia: Lithium to regulate her mood, and antidepressants. Within a few months her supplies were gone, and a family friend who was a doctor prescribed her some new medication. Within a few days of taking these tablets Mum noticed the difference. The mood swings began, where she would veer from manic hysteria to feeling low and lethargic. When we had visitors Mum was loquacious, her voice loud and high-pitched. 'Enough, Fatima,' my grandfather would snap, his dark eyebrows perched on his forehead.

When Mum was well my grandfather only needed to look at her with anger and she would be filled with fear, but as the mania took over she was brave and defiant. Soon my grandparents would send Mum out to run errands when visitors came.

Dido became suspicious that Mum was switching out her medication. He organised Mum's pills in a pillbox and made her take them in front of him. After she'd swallowed the pills with water, she had to open her mouth so he could check that she hadn't hidden any under her tongue or against her cheek, but even with the regular consumption these new pills did not work.

When the mania took hold Mum became boisterous and generous. Before returning to Bosnia Mum had been transferred to a disability pension. Everyone already thought that anyone in Australia was well-off, and the fact that Mum received a pension only reinforced the impression. Since we'd arrived, Mum had relatives coming to my grandparents' house asking to borrow outfits to go out. Mum lent her things to anyone who asked, and soon they even stopped asking. There were times when she'd return to her bedroom to find her clothes had been rifled through. When she asked my grandmother she'd say that somone had come by to borrow Mum's clothes and she'd just told them to help themselves. Sometimes the clothes were returned, sometimes not.

After the woman brought Mum back from her shopping spree Dido checked her bank accounts and found them empty. Some of the recipients of Mum's manic generosity returned the gift bags to her parents; others were not so honest, and kept the money they had 'borrowed' and the 'presents' she had given them.

Dido walked Mum to the hospital and she was admitted to the psychiatric ward. The first thing she noticed when she walked into the hospital ward was the thick cloud of smoke that hung halfway into the room from the ceiling. While smoking was prevalent in all public spaces, Mum was still shocked at the strong smell of tobacco that greeted her. She would soon find out that smoking was one of the few recreational activities permitted in a Bosnian psychiatric hospital.

Mum met Radojka the first day she was there. Radojka, a

university graduate, had a privileged job as a secretary. Her life seemed to be going well, and yet a deep well of depression was pulling her under. One day she'd found herself on the bridge over the Sava River and jumped. She'd been saved by two men who went into the water after her, and that's how she'd found herself in the hospital.

Having Radojka made Mum's stay bearable. Unlike in an Australian hospital, there were no recreational activities available to allow patients to pass the time – not even chess or card games, which were almost national institutions. While there was a television, it was only turned on at night. Instead, patients spent the daylight hours sitting in the recreation room, talking and smoking.

Mum spent her days watching the patients, and while there were a few of them who suffered from a mental illness like her and Radojka, most of them seemed to be fully functional and were treated differently by the nurses on duty.

Mum was to find out that most of the patients sharing the ward with her were in hospital to manage their alcohol-withdrawal symptoms. When heavy drinkers stop abusing alcohol, their previously suppressed neurotransmitters rebound, resulting in brain hyper-excitability. While under the effects, patients can suffer from hallucinations, seizures and delirium tremens, or even die.

In the hospital these patients received benzodiazepines to help them manage the symptoms of their withdrawal. The doctors and nurses were ill-trained to deal with true psychiatric patients.

In an Australian hospital Mum had had regular appointments with a psychiatrist who evaluated her condition and the effects of the medication she was prescribed. Here it seemed the doctors adopted a one-size-fits-all approach. The doctors only appeared on the ward to decide whether a patient would be discharged or remain in hospital; their diagnostic tools were a glance and a brief conversation with the nurses.

Tetka and Tetak visited Mum every day, bringing coffee and food so that she wasn't at the mercy of the hospital's meagre servings: breakfast was a slice of bread and a cup of tea, and the other meals were small portions made from substandard produce. Their visits were only for one hour, so for the other twenty-three hours she was a prisoner in Bedlam.

The first time she went to the toilet there Mum retched as she observed the faeces caked on the wall. There were two toilets for twenty patients and no cleaners regularly checking and cleaning the area or replenishing the toilet supplies. When the toilet paper ran out, patients wiped themselves with their hands and wiped their hands on the wall.

Male and female beds were segregated. The bedsheets were musty, stained and creased: they were changed once a month. Only cold water was available for showers because of a long-debunked medical theory that hot water stimulated the senses.

Within two weeks Mum began to return to my grandparents' house for weekend visits. My brother and I would sleep with her in the middle of the fold-out bed, revelling in Mum's attention, but every Monday Mum was ripped away again to return to hospital. We comforted ourselves that she would be home soon. And she was: after a one-month stay the doctors released her and once again Mum was free to live a normal life.

What Mum didn't realise was that this was the beginning of a cycle: every time my grandparents found her mood swings unmanageable they would admit her to hospital. Under Yugoslavia's Communist regime, people who were different from the so-called 'norm' were viewed as dangerous and were often locked up in institutions. While we lived in Bosnia Mum was incarcerated in hospital whenever she demonstrated the tiniest indication of her illness.

After that first hospital stay I was her only daily visitor, arriving at four o'clock when visiting hours began. Mum spent the day watching the door, waiting for me and my blue hat with the red rose that she had bought at a market. Every once in a while family and friends would drop in, but these visits were sporadic and nothing Mum could depend on.

In the next two years she would be admitted six times, each time for at least a month, sometimes nearly two months. During one of her admissions Mum was reunited with Radojka. Her friend sat in the corner of the room, mute, staring blankly at everyone around her. After Radojka had been discharged she went home and back to work, but her mother confiscated her pay, claiming that Radojka couldn't be trusted. With her independence gone, Radojka gave up and lost hope for the future.

My mother was facing the same predicament. Our family had begun peppering her with advice about what she should do next. While everyone's advice was different, they all agreed on one thing: she should remain in Bosnia and give my brother and me a stable childhood. To do this, they said, she should sell our house in Australia and use the money to build a house on a plot of land next to my grandparents' house that my grandfather had given her. Mum's disability pension would allow her to live comfortably in Bosnia for the rest of her life, and we would be taken care of in the bosom of our family. Mum realised that if she followed this advice she would be at the complete mercy of her family, a fate she began to fear.

By her sixth and last stay Mum understood Radojka. She felt herself freefalling into a depression with no end. She heard the whisper of the Grim Reaper calling to her, telling her that death was the only place that she would be free. In all her times of illness she had never contemplated suicide, but now she was scared by how much death appealed to her. She couldn't take this life anymore. Coming home to Bosnia was supposed to be an oasis; instead it was a prison. She had to escape and return home, back to Australia, and this was how my stepfather entered the picture.

THE BACHELOR

It is a truth universally acknowledged that a single woman with a mental illness must be in want of a husband, to facilitate her escape from familial domination. Thus my thirty-three-year-old mother embarked on her search for a new partner. As in most marriages of convenience, she sought eligible candidates through her networks, and after a few discreet conversations with acquaintances it was her former high school friend, Zlatan, who recommended Izet. Zlatan owned a bakery, which he'd named after himself. 'He's one of my best workers,' Zlatan told Mum. 'He makes pita with a pastry so thin it melts in your mouth. He's lived in Bosanska Gradiška all his life.'

Izet was single and had never been married, which considering that he was thirty-two was quite a feat. Zlatan arranged for Mum and Izet to meet at the annual fair, a travelling carnival set up on council land near the main road. Zlatan had told Izet that Mum was a single mother of two children. Mum had determined that this would be a good first date to test out how child-friendly he was.

She had high hopes: after all, she had met my father during a blind date arranged by family friends. In the year since her divorce Mum had found a job in a factory, where she worked for eleven hours a day and had a few Australian boyfriends. Aida and Zlatan decided to bring her back into the Bosnian fold and arranged a blind date with Hasim, who had migrated to Australia just a few months before.

When my mother opened the front door to greet my father, she was disappointed. He was standing in the bright sun, and as he squinted his crow's feet made him look much older than his twenty-five years.

Mum showed him in, taking a deep breath in anticipation of a torturous night ahead of her. She'd committed to dinner and had to see it through. Behind her, Aida and Zlatan were greeting Hasim. Mum turned around and contained a gasp – he was like a Bosnian Robert Redford with blue eyes and thick blond hair.

After dinner my father drove her home, kissing her deeply at every red traffic light. By the end of the night her face was red from his raspy beard and her lips swollen from his bruising kisses. He made her feel like she was in a romantic movie. In a daze, she didn't realise until he turned off the car that he had driven her to his flat. She went inside with him and he tried to get her into the bedroom.

'No.' She pushed him away. 'I'm not here for that.'

'Then why are you here?' he snapped.

'Take me home now or I'll get a taxi.' Mum headed for the door – an empty bluff since her purse was in his car. She was stranded. Thankfully he walked out after her, banging the front door shut.

As he pulled up in front of her house he said, 'I won't be denied a second time.'

Mum looked at him and her heart danced. He was so handsome. He stared out the windscreen as he gripped the steering wheel, and didn't turn to kiss her goodnight. She got out of the car and watched as he drove off, leaving skid marks as he turned the corner.

On their second date my father brought her straight back home after dinner and they ended up in the back seat. They were having sex when headlights lit up the car. My father had parked halfway across the neighbour's driveway. He quickly yanked up his pants and climbed over the front seat and moved the car. After the neighbours had gone into the house, he climbed back. The mood was ruined for Mum, but he was a man and wanted to finish, so she let him.

They moved in together a few months later and had a housewarming party at their flat in Brunswick. The house was full of Bosnian friends they had made in Melbourne.

One of the older women pulled my father aside. 'You can't do this,' she told him. 'You can't live together in sin. She's already a divorced woman and her reputation will be ruined.'

My father nodded and forced a smile. 'Thank you for telling me.'

Mum was walking into the living room with a tray of drinks when my father called for everyone's attention.

'I have a happy announcement to make.' He smiled.

Mum waited with everyone else, wondering what the announcement could be.

'Fatima and I invited you all here today to tell you that we will be getting married.'

Mum's tray wobbled and she nearly dropped the drinks.

'How wonderful,' someone said.

'Congratulations.'

As Mum received hugs from wellwishers she looked across

the crowd at my father. He was smiling joyfully, acting as if this had been their plan all along.

'What was that about?' Mum asked when she returned from walking the last of the guests out.

'One of those old biddies stuck her nose into my business and started chastising me about ruining your good reputation.' He looked like a pugilist about to enter the ring.

'So you don't want to get married?' she asked.

'No, I do. Of course I do,' he said, sounding like a fervent fiancé. 'I just didn't think it would happen so soon.' While he was furious at the interference, he was also well aware of the proper order of things and wouldn't allow anything to undermine his reputation as a respectable Bosnian man.

In the wedding photos they are a striking couple. Mum is pretty: milky white skin, green eyes, dark wavy hair. She is smiling, her cheeks pink and her face full of hope. Aida had made her a baby-blue wedding dress – after all, she wasn't a virginal bride – with a fitted waist and an A-line skirt. She wore a long lace veil that framed her face and trailed down her back, and held a white posy.

My father looks handsome in a cream suit with thick lapels and flared pants. He wore a rose-patterned tie and white shirt. His dark blond hair shines and he looks seriously at the camera, playing the part of the brooding hero for his beguiling bride.

It seemed that all her dreams were finally coming true. She was living out a fairytale romance.

Now, as my mother waited by the dodgem cars, she could only hope that this blind date would yield a better outcome. She craned her neck looking for Zlatan and Izet, who she'd agreed to meet at seven o'clock, while my brother and I shrieked madly on the dodgems. After three rides we were eyeing our next attraction: the Spire of Death, a cone-like structure where men on motorcycles built up speed until they were riding their bikes against the walls, while the audience stood on the platform above and watched on agog.

We ran Mum ragged over the next two hours as we begged for candy, fairy floss and rides while she slowly relinquished hope that Izet would ever show. As we trudged home that night Mum's feet were heavy with fatigue and she felt the bitter taste of defeat. She had clocked up yet another dud.

The next day Mum went to Zlatan's bakery. 'Where were you?' she demanded.

'I couldn't come,' Zlatan told her. 'Izet went by himself and he was looking for you. He was approaching women who had two children with them, but they looked at him like he was a weirdo so he had to stop.'

Mum sighed and shook her head. Why had she thought this plan would work?

'He really wants to meet you,' Zlatan said, noticing Mum's scepticism. 'Just stay here. I'll get him now.'

Mum sat at the table and waited. She was nervous and full of trepidation, wondering whether she should leave. After all, if they were meant to meet, they would have met the night before.

Zlatan appeared with a man in tow. When Mum caught sight of Izet, she was disappointed. It was true, he was tall, had dark hair and was well-built, but his hairline was receding and he had a very prominent nose. Their eyes met through the window. There was gentleness in his gaze; he looked like a spooked stag. Mum decided to let their meeting play out.

Zlatan served them coffee and they made awkward small talk. Mum knew that she should try to engage in conversation, but she was feeling the pull of lethargy. It was like there were two dogs fighting a war within her: one of them was manic and always barking, while the other just wanted to stretch out by a hearth and sleep. Today lethargy won.

'Say something,' Izet said.

Mum looked at him blankly. 'You say something.'

And so they passed an hour of companionable silence. Mum liked that he was shy, and didn't speak unless he was asked directly. Men of her experience were blowhards who talked and only saw her as a prop for their performance.

'Did you arrange to meet again?' Zlatan asked, as he collected their coffee cups.

'Why should we?' Izet said. 'We just saw each other.'

Zlatan shook his head and looked at Mum with apology in his eyes, but he need not have worried. What Mum liked most about Izet was that he was honest and had no pretensions.

'I'll be here at three o'clock tomorrow,' Izet said as Mum got up to leave.

'I'll see you then.'

When Mum got home she shared the news with her parents that she was going on a date.

'I haven't heard of him,' my grandfather said when Mum told him it was Izet Sakić. 'Maybe your brother will know him. *Stara*, call Raif.'

My grandmother went to the back room and yelled out the window, which faced onto my uncle's part of the property.

Within a few minutes my Dajđa was in the living room.

'Sakić. I know him. The family is poor. There are five children and they all live in a one-bedroom house.'

'Yes, he already told me that,' Mum said.

Izet still lived at home with his parents and a brother, a normal state of affairs in Bosnia where offspring remain at home until they are married; even after matrimony they move in with the husband's parents until they have built their own house, a path my uncle had followed himself.

'Why would you go out with him?' Dajđa asked. 'He works as a baker and doesn't have anything.'

'He is kind,' Mum said.

'The only reason he wants to go out with you is because he's hoping for a ticket to Australia,' Dajđa said.

What my uncle didn't realise was that this was what Mum was banking on. She knew she wasn't much of a marital prospect, but her connection to Australia made her desirable. Izet wanted exactly what she wanted: a new life and a new place to remake himself.

'Let's not be hasty. We have to give him a chance,' my grandfather said. 'All that matters is that he's good to you.'

Mum smiled and left the room. When she returned from the bathroom she overheard my grandfather and Dajđa. Dajđa was calling Izet a pauper and a gold digger.

In the hallway Mum waited to hear my grandfather defend her. 'It's better that she's with him,' Dido said, 'than that she's single and going through different men.'

Mum gasped and left the house. She didn't care if they heard her walking away and realised that she'd been eavesdropping. She couldn't wait to escape and go back home: home to Australia.

Over the next month my mother and Izet embarked on their courtship. Mum was used to men being aggressive and demanding in their expectations of sex, but the most Izet would do was hold her hand. She was worried that he didn't find her attractive, so one day as they were walking to the cinema she cornered him in a doorway and kissed him. When he returned her kiss, she felt relief.

After watching the movie they walked to a cafe to have cake. Izet was even more quiet than usual, but by now Mum had learnt to enjoy the silence and didn't feel obliged to fill it with nonsense chatter.

'I've never been married,' Izet finally said. 'If I wanted to marry you, how would I ask you?'

Mum smiled as delight filled her. Still, she was stumped by his question. She'd never thought about a proposal. Her two other marriages had been decided for her and this was the first time that she was the one doing the choosing. 'You go and ask my father for my hand,' she said, joking.

He nodded and escorted her home. He asked to meet her parents and they arranged a visit that weekend.

Mum spent the day cleaning the house and preparing dinner, under my grandmother's demanding tutelage. Everyone was full of anticipation, but none more than Mum.

At six o'clock Mum heard knocking at the door. 'I'll get it,' Haris shouted and started running, and I followed. Mum ran after us and when we opened the door, Izet stood there, looking bashful. Mum brought him inside and performed introductions.

We sat down to dinner. My grandfather was verbose and Izet mostly nodded. Mum served pita, spiral-shaped pastry that she had helped bake, while my grandmother brought the bowl of *lukmira* salad, diced spring onion in sour cream.

Izet lifted the pita in his hand and looked closely at the pastry. 'It's a nicely formed pita.' He was giving a compliment – he worked in a bakery and made pita for a living – but Nana saw this is a critique of her baking and her face soured.

'I love *lukmira*.' Izet lifted the bowl to his nose and sniffed; the only noise in the now quiet room was his deep inhalation.

Mum had noticed his predilection for smelling his food before he ate and had become used to this eccentricity, but Nana looked at the bowl with disgust and Dido's eyebrows were furrowed over his face.

'It smells delicious,' Izet declared and tipped some onto his plate. Mum took the bowl from him and served herself some and passed the bowl to my nana, who refused to touch it. Dido quickly took it and put some *lukmira* on his plate, where it remained for the rest of the meal.

Dinner passed with Izet oblivious to his faux pas. Afterwards Mum walked him out, and when she returned to the living room Nana was already in the process of cleaning, muttering under her breath about Izet's bad manners and lack of etiquette. As Mum carried the dishes to the kitchen she saw the uneaten salad in the rubbish bin, a waste that was tantamount to a sin to my frugal grandmother.

'Enough, *Stara*,' Dido said, cutting off her tirade. 'He is eccentric, but a suitable match.' Mum did not feel mollified by this. She knew that he thought Izet was the best she could aspire to with her limited prospects.

Mum and Izet began the process of applying to get married, but Dajđa went to see the registrar and told him my mother was mentally ill and that Izet was marrying her only for her money. Dajđa was acting out of concern for my brother and me. We had told our family about what life was like for us before we came to Bosnia: about Mum's frequent hospitalisations and the strangers and family friends who cared for us. They shared our concern that our life would return to the same chaos.

Mum was told that she could only get married if a doctor confirmed that she was of sound mind. After she was examined and had explained the stresses that led to her illness, the doctor recommended the marriage go ahead, but said that Mum shouldn't have any more children because she had had a breakdown every time she'd given birth. Mum felt nothing but relief. A part of her had reservations about this marriage, and the thought of having another a child with her third husband seemed unseemly.

Afterwards Mum asked Izet how he felt about not having a child. 'But I do,' he said. 'Amra and Haris are going to be my children.' Mum didn't know whether he really was sincere, but the fact that he had said it was enough. When they returned to Australia she would have her tubes tied.

My mother and stepfather were married a month later on 7 February 1987. It was a blustery and cold day, so wearing a dress was out of the question. Mum wore her best finery: her knee-high black leather boots, black leather pants and a leather jacket. Izet wore pleated pants, a shirt and a black leather jacket. There was no one to take photos of the event.

Living with my grandparents was out of the question – even if they had invited Mum and Izet to take one of the spare bedrooms, Mum was determined to refuse, as Nana's vitriol and Dido's temper would be a danger to Mum's new marriage.

It was too costly to rent a house for the four of us, and after all, the newlyweds wanted some privacy. When my Dinca told Mum about a friend who had a summer room to rent (the summer room was where the family would cook their meals on a wood-fired stove so the house didn't become too hot), Mum knew she had found their new home. They walked to the wedding registry together and went home as husband and wife.

Mum and Izet moved into the summer room, which was less than three metres wide and had no plumbing. Mum had to pump water from the outside water pump and have buckets of water inside for them to drink and to use for their ablutions. When they wanted to bathe they had to boil the water in a ten-litre copper pot on the wood-fired stove and then pour the water into a tin bathtub. The outside toilet was three metres away.

The only bonus was that the room was already furnished: it had a wooden cupboard where they stored their clothes and foodstuffs that didn't require refrigeration, a fold-out sofa and a small dining table with two chairs. They only had to bring their clothes and they had officially moved in.

They soon settled into a routine. Izet woke at five-thirty in the morning and would quietly perform his ablutions and dress himself and leave for work at six o'clock. Mum remained in bed until nine. After eating breakfast she walked to the *granap* and bought potatoes and ingredients for a stew.

Mum then walked to my grandparents' and had a mid-morning coffee with Nana before preparing dinner for us all, and then took Izet's dinner to the summer room and waited for him to come home around 3 p.m.

Izet was generous with his compliments and appreciated everything Mum did. While life without modern amenities was hard, the fact that Mum knew it was temporary made it bearable. They were organising the paperwork for Izet to get a visa so they could return to Australia together, a laborious process that would end up taking seven months.

One of the things that Mum most appreciated about Izet was his honesty. He would never take money from her purse, even when she asked him to; instead he would hand over her handbag and wait for her to give him money. When he returned from shopping he would place the receipt on the table and carefully stack the change on top of it. After years of being taken for granted by people who saw her pension as free money they could benefit from, Mum finally felt respected and safe.

Haris and I used to spend evenings with Mum and Izet, and when it was time to go home Izet would walk us through the fields and help us across the canal and into the quarter-acre field that made up my grandparents' backyard. For their one-week anniversary Mum made dinner and a cake to celebrate, and I went with her to the summer room. Haris had the morning shift at school the next day so he stayed home.

We waited for Izet to come home and be surprised by our gesture, but soon four o'clock passed and then five and night came, but he didn't show up.

'Mum, where is he?' I asked.

'I don't know.' Time passed slowly as we watched the clock. There was no television to kill time so I started running up and down the street and returning every five minutes to say he wasn't coming. Eventually I tired of the game and quietened on the couch.

'What if something happened to him?' I asked.

'Somebody would come and tell us.'

There was no phone in their room, but we lived in a small village and someone would have come to find Mum if Izet had been hurt. At nine o'clock we walked back to my grandparents' house.

'What are you doing here?' asked Nana.

'Izet didn't come home,' I said, and went to my bedroom.

'I knew that pauper was up to no good,' Nana hissed.

Mum slept with us again that night and she agreed to lie in the middle, with Haris and me on either side of her.

The next morning Mum went to the bakery. Izet looked at her and quickly looked away. She walked up to him and waited. His hands were capably shaping soft dough. 'I won't go back to that room,' he said without looking at her.

She watched his hands, stupefied for a moment as she realised that was all he was going to say. 'You don't have to,' she said and left.

'What happened?' Nana demanded.

'He's not coming back.'

'I knew it. I knew he was a pauper. You should never have married him,' Nana crowed.

Mum was broken, unable to muster a defence. She'd thought her escape was imminent; now all she could see in her future was darkness.

'*Zaveži Stara*,' Dido said, taking a deep drag of his cigarette, his face drawn in lines of sadness. He was disappointed that his black sheep daughter wasn't going to get the image makeover he was so desperate for.

Mum moved back in with my grandparents. A week later

she was on her way to the doctor when she heard someone calling her name. Mum turned around and saw her errant husband. She'd passed by the bakery, forcing herself to walk straight and proud just in case he was inside and watching.

'I would speak to you, if you're not embarrassed to be seen with me.' Izet pointed to his work clothes.

'I'm not embarrassed.'

'I want to get back together.'

Mum knew she should hesitate, make him sweat it out as he wondered whether she would take him back, but she didn't have the heart to pretend. 'I'll see you at home tonight.'

After her appointment, Mum returned to my grandparents' house laden with groceries. When she told her parents that Izet was coming back to her she said, 'I started eating Izet's shit, so I might as well eat it all up.'

When Izet came home from work that night she served dinner as usual. 'What happened?' she asked after he finished eating. When silence greeted her question, she asked again, 'Why did you leave?'

He shrugged and began collecting the dishes, taking them outside to the pump to wash. He never did give her a reason, and she stopped asking. Instead, they settled into an uneven truce, pretending it didn't matter that he left.

GEOGRAPHY

Seka and I became friends because of proximity. She lived three houses away from my grandparents' house. She was one year older than me and we didn't go to the same school, so we only played together at home. Soon after we became friends she came to visit while Haris and Dido were out. Nana served us dinner and we ate on a cloth on the floor. As I bent forward to help myself a fart escaped. I looked at Seka and Nana. They hadn't heard it. I breathed a sigh of relief and kept eating.

'That Seka is so uncouth,' Nana complained when Seka left. 'I don't know how her parents raised her, but it's rude to fart during dinner.'

'It wasn't –' I started to interrupt with my confession.

'I don't want her in my house again,' Nana said as she collected dishes.

My eyes widened. What would Nana say if she knew it was me? I was too scared to find out.

Nana was a judgemental woman, prone to hasty first impressions that never shifted, and she used Seka's infraction to identify her character flaws. According to Nana's ledger Seka was unworthy to play with.

I learnt not to ask for permission to play with Seka, because it wasn't forthcoming. When I tried to get Mum's permission she told me that I had to heed my grandmother and her rules as it was her house. I was on my own.

Nana was in the kitchen. We had a wood-fired stove that warmed up the whole kitchen and living room when she cooked in summer. Nana would be red-faced and sweaty as she stood above the stove. While she was occupied I sneaked through the living room doorway and down the hall. When I got to the front door I crouched down and hugged the wall so Nana wouldn't see me through the windows. I cut across our neighbours' front yards, hiding behind hedges and greenery. If I went down the road Nana would be able to come out of the house and spot me, and once she did I wouldn't be able to pretend I hadn't heard her calling me back. When I got to Seka's house I knew I was safe. Nana wouldn't come to claim me back – after all, what excuse could she use without starting gossip in the neighbourhood?

A balcony jutted out the front of Seka's house next to the living room and the kitchen. The balcony had no fence and it was our usual play area because it allowed us to jump up and down as we pleased. Seka wanted us to make perfume. We got a bunch of cleaning products and vegetables from the garden and began blending them together.

Seka was selective in her approach. She'd add things one drop at a time, sniffing, trying to ensure that her ingredients actually melded into a concoction resembling perfume. I had no such process. I threw things together, enjoying the way different colours melded together and the tactile sensation of squishing cucumber between my fingers, mixing in cleaning products until my container foamed and overflowed. I put on a lid and began shaking it. When I was satisfied that it had mixed together I took the lid off and took a deep whiff. The odour was repugnant. I flinched as the vapours drifted up my nose, making me dizzy and my vision swim. I quickly lay down before I fell.

'Are you okay?' Seka's face appeared above my head.

'I don't feel too well.' I held my stomach, nausea churning, and I swallowed trying to keep it down.

'I'm nearly finished with my perfume and I wanted you to try it.'

'No, no,' I gasped, the thought of sniffing anything else nearly making me vomit. 'I have to go home.'

I jumped off the edge of the balcony. I turned back to wave at Seka, but she was already immersed in making her perfume, her face full of concentration as she tipped in a few drops and took a careful sniff.

'What's wrong with you?' Nana demanded when I got home and carefully sat on the couch.

'Nothing.' I clutched my stomach and leaned my head back.

'What did you eat?'

'Nothing.' I was too weak to shake my head and my voice was barely audible.

'Where were you?' she asked.

I didn't answer.

'Were you playing with Seka?'

I kept myself still.

'I knew it. That Seka gave you something to eat that's making you sick. I'm going to have a talk with her mother.'

'No, no. We were making perfume.'

'What?'

I explained to Nana that we'd been making perfume and the smell had made me sick.

'That Seka is bad news. I told you that.' Nana handed me some mint tea. 'Maybe now you'll believe me and stop playing with her.'

I didn't say anything as I sipped the tea. I wasn't going to make promises that I didn't intend to keep.

During summer the trees in the neighbourhood groaned with fruit. This was the time of year when the village children were seen as useful rather than nuisances to be shooed away. Our tree-climbing skills meant that we were the only ones who could climb to the top and pick all the ripe fruit.

Seka's next-door neighbour offered us the job of picking his plums. Our payment was to eat as many as we wanted while we were picking. There were four of us: Seka and me, and her elder brother Hakija and his friend.

We spent a good hour among the branches, gorging ourselves as we slowly filled up the plastic bags dangling from our wrists. The tree was so bountiful that even though we could hardly move from eating so much, we carefully climbed down with one overflowing plastic bag each.

When I got home Nana had lunch ready, but I shook my head, unable to eat another bite. 'I'm full.'

'What did you eat?' Nana asked.

'We were picking fruit.'

'Who?'

'Seka and me.'

'Was her brother there?'

'Yes.'

'So it was just the three of you?' Nana asked.

'No, Hakija's friend was there too.'

'You shouldn't be playing with boys,' Nana said. 'That Seka might not care about her reputation, but I know what happens when boys and girls play together. You are not to go there again.'

I didn't argue. I knew a futile fight when I heard one. Instead I just quietly sneaked away the next day. We were supposed to be picking fruit again.

When I returned home hours later Nana was in the front yard picking grapes. She saw me cutting across the neighbour's front yard and knew I was returning from Seka's house. 'I told you not to go.' She bent down and picked up a rock. I began to run. She threw the rock. Her throw was to the side and the rock missed me, but I wasn't taking any chances. I retreated to my Dajđa and Dinca's and stayed there for a few hours, quietly sneaking back to my grandparents' house when it was dark. Nana glared as she served me dinner, but nothing more was said.

Years later I spoke to Mum about Nana's prejudice against Seka. 'How could she be so terrible and not allow me to play with her?'

'It wasn't that she didn't want you to play with Seka,' Mum explained. 'It's that she didn't want you to go to Seka's house because of her older brother. Nana was old-fashioned and knew how easily a girl's reputation was ruined.'

Nana's fears were born from hard-earned experience, and if she had shared them with me I would have understood. I had learnt soon after we arrived in Bosnia how precarious life was for an unaccompanied female.

Nana regularly sent me to the *granap* to buy her groceries. A *granap* was usually on the ground floor of the owner's house and there was no such thing as self-serve: you went in with a list and pointed to items on the floor-to-ceiling shelves. I loved going to the *granap* because I was allowed to buy myself a treat for my troubles. I would either buy *Smoki*, a puffy snack made from cornmeal grits flavoured with peanuts, or chewing gum.

It was a warm summer day and the warm breeze fluttered my skirt against my legs as I walked home down the long stretch of unsealed road. The road was quiet, hardly anyone passing by. I was carrying a plastic bag over my wrist as I laboriously fought the wrapper of my chewing gum. The chewing gum was cylindrical, its cigarette-patterned wrapper stuck tight so I had to tear it off one small peel at a time.

A boy appeared next to me. 'Where do you live?' he asked.

'Down the road.' I waved, not looking at him, still consumed with my wrapper. I was still 500 metres from my grandparents' house. There was only one small farmhouse on this stretch of road, which I'd long since passed.

'Who do you belong to?' he asked, the Bosnian way of identifying family connections.

I gave him my grandfather's name, as he was known by all in the neighbourhood. My eyes were still locked on the chewie, which was five centimetres from my face when I saw the boy fiddling with his zipper. A tingle of awareness nudged into my consciousness, and I finally looked up at his face. He was looking away, his head turning in one direction and then the other like a bird, scoping out if anyone was coming.

'I'd better get going,' I said.

He looked at me and our eyes met. I read his intent in them.

He pushed me to the ground and lay on top of me, holding me down as he tried to lift my skirt. The chewie fell as I fought him, the hard rock of the asphalt pushing into my back.

I fought like a trapped animal, and just as my strength was failing he got off me. He ran off in the direction of my grandparents' house. I stood up shakily, my hands trembling as I scooped up the shopping bag, my feet kicking the chewie further away as I ran back to the *granap*.

Terrified, I stood next to the door of the shop, trembling as I relived the encounter, fearing the boy would come back to find me. After half an hour the shop owner's glare became difficult to ignore and I ventured back out again. I took another route to my grandparents' house, running along the canal, and got there sweaty and feverish. Nana was cross that I had taken so long, but I didn't tell her what happened.

Over the next few days I was terrified to run any of the numerous errands my grandparents passed on to me. In desperation I confided in my cousin when we were alone in her room.

'What were you thinking, you stupid girl?' she lectured. 'You know that you have to keep your eyes open.'

My eyes smarted. She was acting like it was my fault.

'You can't tell anyone,' she said, gripping my hands. 'You know what people are like.' She looked out the window.

I did. The year was 1985 but in Bosanska Gradiška it might as well have been 1955. Attitudes were old-fashioned. Girls had to be modest and careful with their reputations. If they were compromised, even through no fault of their own, they were forevermore seen as damaged goods and would be the source of perpetual gossip.

But Nana never shared her concerns about Seka's brother with me; instead, all I knew as an eight-year-old was that Nana was being horrible to my friend. Our friendship continued in stealth for a few more months, until the incident that ended it forever.

Only the old part of my grandparents' house had a pitched roof; the roof over the newer rooms was flat, and the family used it as an extended balcony. Dido had built steep stairs on the side of the house to allow us to get up there. The stairs had no railing, so I would hold onto the wall as I climbed them, always feeling like I was about to fall off.

During summer I'd go upstairs with the adults, who would drink coffee sitting on a blanket, picnic-style. It was magical to feel the warm concrete beneath me while the breeze cooled me. I loved peering into the neighbours' yards. There was no fence around the edge of the roof and my grandparents warned me to always keep well back.

One day Seka and I were playing and I told her about the view from the roof. 'I've never been,' she said.

'Really?' I said, although I wasn't surprised. My grandparents and her parents didn't really socialise.

'I'd love to see it.'

'I'll show you.'

Seka's eyes narrowed. 'Are you sure?'

'Sure, we can go now,' I said, even though I was expressly forbidden from going upstairs by myself. I figured that as long as my grandparents didn't find out, it wouldn't matter. I was full of bravado and daring, wanting to be the one to show Seka the magical view from the balcony.

We tiptoed through the hedges. When we reached my grandparents' house I left Seka hiding behind a shrub while I sneaked over to check if Nana was in the yard.

It was all clear. I ducked under the kitchen windows and Seka followed. We tiptoed up the stairs and onto the roof. We walked to the edge and looked out.

'It's amazing.' Seka's face lit up with wonder.

I felt a sense of satisfaction. We were a metre away from the edge, as close as my grandparents allowed me to get. I realised that there was no one around to stop me from getting closer. I edged further out.

'Amra, get back,' Seka called.

I ignored her, excited by my daring. Adrenaline surged through me when I reached the edge, the toes of my sneaker touching the gutter.

'Amra, now!' Seka shouted, her voice louder.

I turned around to tell her to shush, scared that my grandparents would hear her. In summer the windows were kept open to let in air and sound travelled from the roof. As I turned my head to look at her, I let go of the edge. I had the sensation of flying and then blackness.

I woke up in hospital eight hours later. I'd fallen two metres off the house, my body smashing onto the concrete below. Tetka and Mum ran out of the house and found me lying there. Tetka scooped me up in her arms and ran to the main road. She flagged down a passing car and they drove me to hospital.

Mum spent all afternoon beside my hospital bed, waiting for me to wake up. The nurses told her visiting hours were over and that she had to leave. She went home and got my favourite doll, a rollerblading doll she'd bought me in Singapore on our way to Bosnia.

When I woke up I couldn't remember anything. I didn't know where I was or why I was there.

'It's okay,' a nurse said. 'You were in an accident and you're in hospital now.'

'Where's my mummy? I want my mummy,' I cried.

'She waited for you to wake up all day, but she had to go home.'

'But I want her. I want Mummy.' I began crying in big gulping sobs.

'She'll be back tomorrow morning.' The nurse handed me the doll. 'She left this for you.'

'I want Mummy.' I was crying as I clutched the doll.

'Stop crying,' the nurse said. 'You're disturbing the other patients.'

I looked around and saw eyes peering at me from the bed next to mine. 'But Mummy,' I said pitifully.

'You'll see her tomorrow. Now go to sleep.'

I cried myself to sleep.

I was in hospital for a few days. A welcoming party of people from the neighbourhood greeted me when I returned home. I walked in, limping because my hip had been hurt when it connected with the concrete. An X-ray had uncovered a slightly loosened hip socket which would continue to plague me as I got older. When I became a teenager I learnt very quickly not to wear high heels or bad footwear, or agonising pain would shoot up my leg.

I enjoyed the attention after my accident. I'd had a lucky escape and everyone knew it. I must have become unconscious on the way down and didn't make any effort to stop my fall. I fell on my side and scraped the whole left side of my face.

I couldn't remember what had happened on the roof. Years later a image appeared in my mind of me on the roof with Seka. The image was like a dream, bleached of colour and sound. In it I turned to look behind me as I crouched close to the edge, and then there was nothing but blackness, until the hospital.

Because I couldn't remember what had happened, there were a lot of questions I couldn't answer. Of course it didn't take long for Nana's suspicions to turn to Seka. 'Where was Seka when you were close to the edge?' she asked.

'Behind me.'

'She pushed you, didn't she?'

'No!' I was shocked. 'Of course not. I fell off when I was too close to the edge.'

'Hmmm,' Nana said, her face telling its own story.

No matter how many times I denied it, Nana had her own version of the truth. I tried sneaking away again to play with Seka, but she was always busy. The rumour mill had done its job and our friendship was over.

The scrape on my cheek became a dark, red scab as it dried. I visited a neighbour, a girl a few years older than me who I admired greatly. She kept staring at the scab. 'I can help you get it off,' she finally said.

'How?' I touched my face self-consciously. My cheek felt like leather, with the scab all dry and rough. I hated having it on my face. People looked at me like I was a freak and wanted to know the why of it all.

'You just peel it.' She reached her hand towards me.

'No!' I jerked away. 'It's going to hurt.'

'No, it won't. Come here and I'll show you.'

Reluctantly I went back and she began scratching at my scab. The first scratch didn't hurt and the scab came off by itself. As she continued, some bits of scab still stuck to the skin and there was a stinging pain.

'Ouch.' I pulled away and covered my face with my hand.

'Here, have a look.' She handed me a mirror.

My skin looked pink and dry as if it was sunburnt. There were bits of blood where the soft new layer of skin had peeled.

'Here, I'll take the rest off.'

I didn't want her to, but the scab looked worse than the peeled skin underneath and so I endured it until the scab had all come off. Afterward I held the dried scab in my hands, touching its wrinkled hardness. The scab was like a mask that I had now taken off, revealing the real me underneath.

I wondered how things would have turned out if I had told Nana it was her granddaughter who was uncouth and had broken wind during dinner. I stroked my finger along the scab's wrinkled hide and threw it in the rubbish bin.

NOT A FAIRYTALE

'What is the movie again?' Mum asked as she poured coffee from the *džezva*, a long-necked coffee pot with a long handle. Izet was taking her to a movie and she was excited to have a night out.

'*One Thousand and One Nights.*' Izet took a sip from the little half-cup.

I was sitting on the couch opposite them and when I heard the movie title my eyes widened with curiosity. 'Can I come?'

'Me too.' Haris rubbed his hands together, looking like he was crumbling feta with them, a motion he always did when he was excited.

The story of Scheherazade was legendary. A sultan is dishonoured by his wife and has her executed. In order to guarantee that he will not suffer infidelity again, he marries a succession of virgins only to execute each bride the next day. Eventually there are no virgins left and the vizier's daughter Scheherazade volunteers to marry the sultan. Scheherazade is very clever and has learnt from all the women who came before her. She asks the sultan if he would like to hear a story and proceeds to tell him a tale that takes all night and has not yet reached its conclusion when dawn lights up the sky. The sultan spares her life so that he can hear the ending. And so the tales continue, for one thousand and one nights, until the Sultan admits his love for Scheherazade and spares her life. I was in love with the fairytale and agog at the chance to see the movie.

'You can come with us next time,' Izet said.

I hid my face with my hair. He was just like all of Mum's boyfriends, full of empty promises.

'Why don't you take the children?' Nana piped up from the kitchen. My grandmother was supposedly cleaning the dishes, while in actual fact she was avoiding Izet. She had nothing but bad things to say about him behind his back, and did her best to not speak to him when he was in her presence.

'It's not a movie for children,' Izet protested.

'Of course it is,' Nana growled. Nana thought he was trying to talk down to her. She was illiterate and had been subjected to a lifetime of put-downs by my grandfather, who demanded her silence.

'This is an adult movie,' Izet tried again, but Nana would give no quarter. She took special relish in browbeating him into acquiescence. Now that Izet was taking Mum out on a date, Nana had found the right moment for revenge for his gaffe the first night he came to dinner. 'It's so sad that the poor child should miss out.' In my grandfather's absence my grandmother could let loose her natural tendency to meddle and manipulate. 'And Scheherazade is Amra's favourite fairytale.'

'I love her so much,' I said, getting in on the act. 'Can I come, please?'

'Please, please,' Haris begged too.

'Look how much they're begging.' Nana glared at Mum. Mum was looking at the floor, pretending this conversation had nothing to do with her, but the fact that she wasn't supporting Izet spoke volumes.

'All right, they can come,' Izet finally said, his head bowed and voice defeated.

As we made our way to the town centre, Izet walked behind as if he was heading to his execution, while Haris and I skipped eagerly ahead. Mum tried to talk to Izet, but he was silent and intractable. It was sundown; the movie session began at eight o'clock, which should have been clue it wasn't for children.

When we arrived there was a line of people stretching to the theatre door. There was only one cinema in town and the movie would play for months, giving everyone the chance to see it at least once. I searched the crowd as we lined up, but Haris and I were the only children. The other adults were looking at us askance. Izet was well known in town from his job at the bakery, and many people greeted him. He nodded silently, not lingering for conversation. His whole posture was one of silent suffering. He'd promised my grandmother that he would take us to see the movie and he saw no way out.

Izet bought tickets from the reluctant sales clerk and we headed inside. It was opening night and every seat was full. The credits rolled and Scheherazade began her first tale, but this was no ordinary fairytale. *One Thousand and One Nights* was an erotic take on the fable and all Scheherazade's stories featured lusty romps and ended with Scheherazade performing a juicy blowjob on the mighty sultan. As she wiped her lips afterwards she said teasingly, 'I'll finish the story tomorrow night,' and sashayed out of the sultan's bedchamber.

Each scene was etched in my mind like a stencil drawing. The first tale was Aladdin and the magic carpet, except Aladdin was no ordinary thief. Instead of jewels or money, he stole women's virtue. He swooped down into a village and watched as a husband left his sleeping wife to go to work. Aladdin snuck into the bedchamber and disrobed. He lay down behind the sleeping woman and with one thrust of his hips, he was inside her, her bedsheet slipping to reveal her bosom. She conveniently kept her eyes closed during the proceedings, supposedly half asleep as she called out her husband's name.

Just as their cries of passion reached a screeching crescendo, the husband returned, calling his wife's name as he walked through the front door. She opened her eyes and saw the stranger who was lying with her and screamed. Aladdin stood, pulled up his pants and ran as the husband chased him. Aladdin jumped out the window and onto his magic carpet and sped away across the bright blue sky, searching for another maiden to ravish.

Even though there were sex scenes, this was the eighties and the movie was soft porn: there were no close-ups of penises, the women's bushes were tastefully trimmed, and the breasts were bouncy and natural.

I was enthralled by the action on the screen. When my brother and I watched movies with my grandparents we had to leave the room and wait in the hallway when the characters exchanged a passionate kiss and we were never exposed to any of the numerous sex scenes in European movies. There were some nights it seemed I was spending more time in the hallway than I was on the couch.

Haris was laughing hysterically and rubbing his hands with glee as he watched the rude bits.

'Stop laughing,' Mum snapped, her hand gripping Haris's arm as heads turned towards us.

His peels of laughter were drawing everyone's attention to

the fact that there were children in the theatre. I began laughing too, and couldn't stop. Realising that she was creating a greater disturbance by shushing us, Mum looked straight ahead and pretended we were not her progeny.

This was the final straw for Izet. He leapt out of his seat and pushed his way to the aisle, his long-limbed stride eating up the stairs. He shoved open the emergency door and let the bright streetlight into the theatre, causing a groan from the audience as it flashed over the screen. His shadow seemed to hang suspended there for a moment, before he disappeared from view and the doors clanged shut behind him.

Mum looked around, and realising that she didn't want to be left behind in enemy territory, she yanked Haris and me out of our seats. As she dragged us down the aisle I kept my eyes on the two-metre screen, watching the back of Scheherazade's head as she performed yet another blowjob on the sultan, his cries of ecstasy spilling past his lips as he clutched her hair.

Izet walked us home, this time walking briskly so that we struggled to keep up with him. When we reached my grandparents' house Mum sent Haris and me inside alone, while Izet impatiently waited on the street. The last thing I saw was her trying to keep up with Izet's strides as he walked home like the hounds of hell were nipping at the soles of his feet.

The next morning I overheard Mum and Nana talking after Dido had left the house.

'There was nudity,' Mum whispered.

'Really?' Nana exclaimed in shock. 'How could that be? It's a children's fairytale.'

Mum shook her head. 'Izet tried to tell you it was for adults only, but you wouldn't listen.'

'You were there too.' Nana was quick to shift the blame. 'You could have spoken up.'

'Izet was embarrassed because everyone was looking at us,' Mum said.

'Well, that's his problem. He shouldn't have taken children to such an inappropriate movie.'

Mum gave Nana a dirty look. Nana was acting as if Izet had had a choice, when in fact she had mercilessly bullied him into it. I wondered why he'd given in and taken us, but I guess there really is no way to tell your mother-in-law that you're planning on taking her daughter to see an erotic movie.

Soon after this Izet's visa came through and my mother was finally able to escape her family's domination, but there was just one problem – my brother and I did not want to return to Australia with her and Izet. She attempted bribery, buying me a pink plastic toy sewing machine that ran on batteries and my brother a racing car, but we held firm. While living with our grandparents came with a price, we had stability and routine, and we were not willing to give it up. Defeated, Mum finally booked their tickets and she and my stepfather left for Australia.

UNSUITABLE FRIENDSHIPS

'Wait here while I talk to my grandmother,' I told my friend Gordana at the front door of my grandparents' house. Gordana had invited me to her home the week before and I'd had the best time. She had her own room and she'd played her guitar for me. I reciprocated by spontaneously inviting her to my house after school without checking with my grandmother beforehand.

'*Šta joj je ime?*' Nana asked me her name.

'Gordana.'

'She's a *Vlah*,' Nana spat out, a rude term that meant she was not Muslim. I glanced behind me. I'd left the door open and Nana was talking loudly. 'She's not coming into my house.'

I wanted to sink through the floor with embarrassment. What was I going to do? I went back outside. Gordana was a few metres away from the house and looking towards the backyard. Maybe she hadn't heard? 'Let's go to the roof.' I took her up the stairs and we sat down and talked. She was too polite to ask why I hadn't invited her in and I was too embarrassed to tell her the truth. She didn't stay long and I learnt that my friendships had to take place away from my grandmother.

Alma was my next friend and she was a wild child like me – her mother worked and her father was out of the picture – so we were wild with freedom to do what we liked. It was winter and so we started hanging around at the shopping centre after school to keep warm. We gravitated towards the confectionary section, where I would hungrily look at the chocolate. I never had any money of my own and chocolate was a luxury that I hardly ever got to eat since Mum had left for Australia.

Alma picked up two chocolates and looked at the wrappers. She lifted her arm up, pretending to point to another shelf, and slid one chocolate up her sleeve before returning the second chocolate to the shelf. She nodded, urging me to do it. I quickly looked around and repeated her sleight of hand. I wasn't as smooth in my technique but the result was the same: I felt the hard edge of the chocolate bar against my arm.

We wandered around a little more, pretending we were looking at other things before we left. As we passed the security guard standing by the entrance my whole body broke out in a nervous sweat and I kept my face down. As soon as we'd reached the park beyond the shopping centre we whooped and cheered.

I got out my 300 gram Mikado chocolate bar and gently caressed the wrapper, which was red with a woman in a kimono. As I ripped it open and bit into the milk chocolate dotted with white rice puffs, I was blissed out on sugar. When I got home my grandparents demanded to know where I had been since school had finished hours ago. I let silence be my weapon.

Soon Alma and I were inseparable. We went to the shops every day and repeated our chocolate collection technique. We weren't the only ones shoplifting. We saw many people stuffing things down their waistbands, or lifting their pants and wedging food items into their boots. For us stealing chocolate was a way of getting a treat we were usually denied, while for others shoplifting was the only way to put food on the table.

By the time we finished eating the whole chocolate bar my stomach would be distended and sore, but there was no way of taking it home to eat later. My grandparents would suspect something.

When I went to the shopping centre with my cousin Safija a few weeks later, I performed my magic trick with two chocolates. Safija's face darkened and she walked away from me, practically running for the door. I followed her with a swagger, feeling pride in my achievement.

'Hey, *mala, prestani*.' A male voice called out to me to stop and a hand grabbed my shoulder.

I turned around, my stomach dropping when I saw it was the security guard.

'Give it.' He gestured with his hand towards my sleeve.

I put my arm down and the chocolate fell into my hand. I handed it over.

'Don't come back here. You're banned.'

He returned to the shopping centre while I ran to my cousin, who was waiting for me across the street.

'What were you thinking?' Safija shouted. 'I had to leave or he'd think I was in on it.'

I wiped away a tear. I'd got away with shoplifting so many times it had become normal for me to take what I wanted. Being caught and shamed was a reality check, and seeing my cousin's disgusted expression I realised how far I'd stepped outside of society's norms.

'What did he say?' she demanded.

'He told me not to come back,' I wailed.

'What did you expect?' Safija snapped. 'You're known to

them as a shoplifter now. Any time you go in you'll be watched or told to leave.'

I began crying in earnest. This was the only shopping centre and now I could never enter it again. I was devastated.

Now that the shopping centre was out of bounds, Alma invited me to her house for lunch after our morning shift at school, while her mother was at work. We were sitting on the sofa and I was looking out the window admiring the blanket of snow that covered everything. Alma had lit a fire in the fireplace and it was getting warm, but it was still too cold for me to take off my green nylon snow suit.

'Do you know what sex is?' Alma asked.

'Of course. A man puts his penis in a woman's vagina.'

Alma looked impressed that I knew the mechanics of the act. 'Have you ever done anything like that?'

I nodded.

'What did you do?'

'A boy took me to his room and he took off our pants. He tried to put his pipi inside me,' I told her. 'But then his mother came and interrupted us.'

'My uncle comes and plays with me while Mum is at work. He takes off our pants and we do stuff.'

'What stuff?'

'Things that grown-ups do.' She shrugged.

'Really?' I was jealous. She made it sound like I'd been robbed by not having Fadil do stuff with me.

'You want me to show you?' she asked.

'Okay.'

'Lie down on the sofa,' she directed me.

I lay on my back, fully clothed. Alma pushed my legs

apart and lay between them. She ground her pelvis against my pelvis. The friction stimulating my clitoris sent shock waves of pleasure through me. It was the first time I'd felt that sort of pleasure and the more she did it, the more it built up. As she closed her eyes her face took on a look of pleasure, and the only sounds in the room were the squeak of my nylon suit and our faint moans.

'It would be better if we had a boy here,' she said. 'Boys have pipis that they put inside you and can make you feel good.'

I felt restless and unsettled. I needed a sense of completion.

'Maybe a boy will come by now and we can call him inside,' Alma said.

We sat up and looked out the window but no one was passing by.

'Let's try some more,' she said. I lay back down and she kept grinding her pelvis against me. 'We should take our clothes off.'

'Really?' I gulped. I wasn't sure that I wanted to try that.

She kept moving her pelvis as she talked. 'Yes, it will feel even better.'

My bowels moved. Whenever I got excited I had to poo. Soon enough the pressure overcame my pleasure and her pressing on my pelvis increased the pressure. 'I have to poo.'

'Really?' She was disappointed as she stopped.

'Really.' I pushed her off and ran to the toilet. I tried to poo, but I was backed up. I was under pressure to finish defecating so I could go back out and play, and the more I tried to poo, the more it retracted back up my colon.

'How long are you going to be?' she called out.

'Not long.' I strained as I tried to push it out.

I stayed in the toilet for at least five minutes, but I was too agitated. All the emotions that were going through me were confusing me. I wanted to go out and play the game with Alma and feel those amazing sensations of pleasure, but I was also scared about the way the game was changing. Eventually I left the toilet and returned without doing a poo. 'I have to go home.'

I wasn't able to defecate anywhere but in my own toilet. This had led to many pains in the abdomen when I held it in at school or when playing, but I'd learnt not to fight my stomach or my bowels after soiling my pants a few months ago.

I'd been playing with Haris and a few friends and we'd been pushing each other in a wheelbarrow. I could feel that I needed to go, but hadn't wanted to stop playing. As I picked up the handles of the wheelbarrow with Haris sitting inside, the strain pushed on my bowels and the poop jumped out of me. I hobbled home, feeling the squishy poo pressing against my skin. I took off my underwear and folded it to hide the poo. After washing myself I snuck outside to the barn and buried the stained undies in the manure pile. I never would have been able to live down being an eleven-year-old who shat her pants.

So now as Alma urged me to go back to the toilet to try again, I knew it was time to go home. My stomach was twisting itself in pain and my colon felt tender so I couldn't sit comfortably. 'No, I've got to go.' I didn't want to risk another accident. I got my backpack and left.

Alma watched me from the window as I trudged through the snow. I waved at her, but she didn't wave back.

When I got home I rushed to the toilet. As my body purged

itself I realised I'd been on the edge and had been saved from disaster. I never went back to Alma's house and our friendship petered out after I refused her invitations to visit again, too scared that her uncle might be in attendance to continue our sexual education.

NEW PLAYMATE

'One, two, three,' I counted under my breath as I two-stepped to the polka in the school gym during PE class. As eleven-year-olds we were of the age where we didn't want to touch the opposite gender, so my schoolmate Gordana was my partner. I had my hands on her shoulders, while she held my waist.

As we twirled among the rest of the class I saw a movement in the doorway. A mascot bear appeared and started dancing. We gathered around to watch as it did backflips in the middle of the gym. I laughed until my stomach hurt. I hadn't been laughing much since Izet and my mother had gone to Australia.

Haris and I had been too afraid of how Mum's hospitalisation would affect us, and so we'd resisted Mum's efforts to convince us to go with them. While I'd had many upheavals during my young life, the one constant had been my mother. Now that she was in another country and completely lost to me, I realised how much she was a part of me. Missing her was like a physical ache that I could not assuage.

The mascot bear stopped dancing and lifted its arms. It removed its head and my mother's smiling face appeared. I ran towards her and she hugged me hard until I couldn't breathe. Everything felt right with the world again.

'Amra, lift those feet,' my gym teacher said, breaking my reverie.

I was once again in the gym dancing with Gordana. In the five months since Mum had gone, I had developed intricate fantasies about her coming back. As I walked home from school I would imagine Mum was waiting from me, until my steps quickened and I ran home, out of breath and sweaty, only find that she wasn't there. As I walked to school I developed fantastical daydreams about the myriad ways that she would surprise me by showing up.

Without Mum around to soften the hard edges, life with Nana and Dido was getting unbearable. There were none of the luxuries that I took for granted with my mum. Mum had bought me low-fluoride toothpaste that was banana flavoured. Nana hid it on the top shelf because it was too expensive to use and so I hardly cleaned my teeth for a while, until the day I found a big chunk of old food between my teeth and realised that I was risking an infection that would necessitate the removal of all my teeth, an affliction that most of my family had suffered from.

Now that Mum had vacated her parental role, my grandmother gained star billing. We watched movies together. At first I translated the American movies into Bosnian for her. As my English skills rusted I instead read the subtitles. My grandmother was illiterate, and before I came along she'd lived most of her life in silence, a witness to my grandfather's storytelling and political diatribes. I became Nana's confidante. The one she told stories to because I listened in rapt silence and awe.

One day, after Dido and Haris had left on the blue tractor, Nana and I went to the shed. She carried outside a small cast-iron stove that we used in summer to cook outside to avoid heating up the house. Nana was known for performing a healing ritual of *salivati stravu* for anyone who needed her help. People with a great terror haunting their sleep, or a terrible disease that had no cure, or a chronic pain that no painkiller would ease, would come to her and she would pour away their fear, sickness or pain using the power of fire and lead. My grandfather didn't approve of the practice because superstition was forbidden in Islam, so Nana could only perform it when he was away from the house.

This ritual was molybdomancy, a divination technique using molten metal dropped into water. The diviner would take out the hardened shape and view it, attempting to divine a message from the other-worldly spirits. My grandfather told me that this ritual had been passed down from our Bogumil ancestors.

On this day I was my nana's subject. The night before I'd had a nightmare about a snake, which according to folklore heralded that I had an enemy wishing me ill will, and so the ritual was required to protect me from the evil eye. I had watched the ritual many times. Nana performed *salivate stravu* for friends and family. She had attempted to cure Mum many times, but to no avail.

Nana sat on a stool in front of the woodstove and I sat next to her. The smoke billowed around us, smoking our clothes. Nana held pieces of lead in her hand, the squares neatly piled on top of each other, the cut edges curling up. She waved her hand around her my head three times while her lips moved with prayer. Nana pulled my T-shirt away from my chest and gave it to me to hold. While I held the bunched up T-shirt with both hands Nana threaded the small lead pieces between my T-shirt and my chest three times. Her lips moved as she recited an Arabic prayer from the Qur'an to herself.

She placed the lead in a metal scoop and put it on the fire to melt, while I sat on a low stool with a red cloth over my head. The red cloth served a practical purpose: to protect my face from stray drops of water, and to ward off the curse of the evil eye. I held a saucepan of water near my head. Nana took the melted lead off the fire. She turned the scoop upside down and dropped the lead into the cold water, making it sizzle and pop. Nana reached into the water and pulled out the lead. She turned the congealed mass in her hand, trying to see a shape in it.

'*Ruža*. A rose,' she muttered under her breath. I waited for Nana to tell me what it meant, but she loved having power and remained silent. She put the lead back into the scoop and placed it on the fire, gripping the handle awkwardly with her clawed right hand. This was a product of Dido's rage years before. He'd been hitting Nana across her back and shoulders with a stick. Nana had lifted her hand to protect her face, there was a crack, and Nana screamed as her fingers broke. The doctor put the fingers in a cast, telling Nana he would take it off in six weeks. The white plaster got cracked and filthy from farm work. A week later Nana yanked the plaster off, and she was left with crooked index and little fingers.

I held the saucepan over my covered legs, the red cloth undulating in the breeze. Nana dropped the lead into the saucepan again. Nana put a cloth over the saucepan to strain out the lead and I tipped the saucepan to my mouth and drank the water. When I lifted my lips the white cloth was stained black.

Nana's mother, Muradija, had taught her the ritual. Muradija had had the touch. She would throw beans to predict events for those wanting to know the future. Her reputation spread so far that a man once came from Croatia to ask her to cure his ailing daughter. Many doctors had performed tests, to no avail. One doctor had told him there was no cure. Muradija cured his daughter by the power of fire and lead. For years afterwards he sent her presents to show his gratitude. Nana told me that she didn't have Muradija's touch, but she knew enough to be able to provide relief to those wanting it.

'My mother, your great-grandmother, had a very hard life,' Nana told me as we sat outside, stirring the cooking pot. 'Muradija became an orphan when both her parents died. She was living with cousins who didn't want to be burdened with another mouth to feed and decided to marry her off, even though she was so young her breasts were like mosquito bites.' Nana held up her hands to her chest and mimed a pinching motion.

'Her husband's family were poor and they all lived together in the one room. Whenever Muradija's husband moved towards her with the intent of consummating the marriage, she would tell him, "I'll scream if you do," and so a few months passed and she was still a virgin.' Nana chuckled as she marvelled at her mother's ingenuity.

'She left her first marriage and met her second husband. He was handsome like a movie star, but she soured on him after their wedding night. He was so rough when he took her, she said that she bled buckets of blood and she could never look at him the same again. And that's when she met my father.'

Nana paused, her eyes looking far away for a moment. 'My father was a wealthy widower. He had a son from his first marriage who was close in age to my mum. She used to tell me stories that they used to play outside in the snow and go sledding together, but soon enough her play stopped when she became a mother.'

My great-grandmother had twelve children, six boys and six girls, and my grandmother was her third child. Nana grew up in relative luxury, but by the time she was adolescent her father had passed away, and the wealth and land her father had accrued were taken by the Communists.

I met my great-grandmother Muradija only once, when we visited Bosnia when I was five years old. With her prominent nose and her tiny cottage. I was convinced she was a witch and would eat me, like she was straight out of Hansel and Gretel. I refused to go to her, even though she begged for a hug.

Muradija lived into her nineties and died in relative poverty. 'But she had a good death,' Nana said. 'God took her while she was sleeping, which is the best death anyone could ask for.'

Nana's eyes teared up. She'd spent the last few years of her mother's life running outside first thing in the morning, peering down the road towards Muradija's one-bedroom cottage, trying to see whether smoke was coming from the chimney. The day her mother died there had been no smoke and she'd felt her heart lurch. 'When I found her she was lying on her side, her hand under her cheek, a smile on her face as if she knew that she was going to heaven.' Nana wiped away a tear as she stirred the pot. She loved telling me stories about her mother, and I loved listening to her.

Every day as I walked home from school I always stopped to look in the window of a lovely clothes shop. When Mum had been with us in Bosnia there was a chance that I could get one of the garments I admired, but now all I could do was peer inside with a sick feeling of envy in my stomach.

There was no school uniform so children wore whatever clothes they had. You knew how much money their parents had by their clothes. My friend Sanela lived in a high-rise and her parents were professionals. She always had beautiful clothes and I hated her for it. Then there was Ana who lived on my street. Her father worked in a factory and her mum stayed at home. She wore threadbare tracksuit pants that stretched and sagged.

I started school looking exotic in my clothes from Australia: new jeans, lovely jumpers and pretty summer dresses. As time passed Mum replaced these with clothes from Bosnia. While I didn't have a plentiful wardrobe, Mum had still bought me good-quality clothes. When I outgrew my clothes after Mum left, replacements were slow to come. Soon I was wearing cheap tracksuit pants and had no jeans to wear.

Mum and I wrote letters to each other and I would sit at the kitchen table and pen my missives, with Nana adding notes.

'Tell her to send money to buy you jeans,' Nana said. I didn't know it at the time, but my mother sent money every month, and a good amount, but Dido took this money and deposited it in the bank, leaving Nana struggling to stretch the meagre amounts he gave her for household expenses as well as clothing me and Haris.

Soon Nana began dictating my letters to Mum, getting more and more verbose about my stepfather and his unsuitability.

She knew that Dido would never approve of what she was telling me to write – he was glad that Mum was married to Izet, and not on the prowl for a husband – so we retreated to a paddock a few houses away, where we sat on a blanket.

'Tell her that she could have married someone better. That if she'd walked to a market and picked the first man she ran into, he would have been better than that pauper.' Nana waited until I'd finished writing and then asked me to read it back to her, giving her the chance to check that I was writing down word for word what she'd said.

Nana got caught up in having her own personal secretary to give her a voice she'd never had before. She had never had the freedom to express her opinions without a filter, and the power went to her head.

Soon Nana expected me to spend all my time with her, either as a friend or a helpmate, and I had to sneak away to play with my friends. When I returned hours later she'd give me the silent treatment.

The morning after one of my sneaky play dates I woke up to a sound I didn't recognise and opened the bedroom door to see my grandmother sweeping the hallway. She was bent over, using a broom with a broken handle that barely reached up to her knees. The exertion must have caused agonising pain through her back and legs, but she stoically swept.

She heard the door open and turned to look at me. I recognised the anger on her face: she was furious. 'Nana, do you want me to help?' I asked as I stood beside her. She continued sweeping as if I hadn't spoken. 'Here, let me take over.' I reached for the broom. She turned away from me and continued.

I went to the kitchen and made myself breakfast. Usually it was waiting for me. This was her way of expressing her rancour. She ignored me for the whole day, so I was forced to follow her around like a lost puppy, begging for the moment when she would once again deign to acknowledge me. She never said why; I had to figure it out. In this instance I should have woken by myself and started helping her with housework. Instead of waking me, she just got on with it and gave me payback.

My grandparents had old-fashioned views of life and of child-rearing. Being a child of 1980s Australia, I always seemed to be out of touch with their idea of propriety. I snuck away to a friend's house and we put nail polish on each other's nails. I was so happy to look down at my hands and see the pink colour gleaming, making my hands look elegant and my fingers long. When I arrived home I showed Nana. 'Do you like my nail polish?'

Even though she would criticise young women who passed by the house wearing short skirts or make-up, calling them tarts, a few months earlier she had revealed her secret desire. We had been watching television when Nana left the room. No one looked up, assuming she'd gone to the toilet. An inordinate amount of time passed.

'Where is Nana?' Dido asked.

I shrugged, engrossed in the television.

'Go find her,' Dido said.

I gave him a dirty look, annoyed, but I knew better than to argue with that voice. I opened the door to the hallway and went to the bathroom. She wasn't there. I looked through each of the bedrooms – they were empty.

The door to the second living room was closed. This was the special living room, which had a lovely, brand-new couch that was hardly ever sat on and a wall unit that covered the whole wall and was used to store all sorts of knick-knacks.

I opened the door. Nana looked up. She was going through my mother's make-up and had found the blue eyeshadow. She was holding a mirror as she dabbed it on her eyelid.

I began laughing and ran to the living room. 'You've got to see this,' I cried out. Dido and Haris followed me. Nana was sitting where I'd left her. She knew she couldn't hide the inevitable. She had a sheepish smile on her face.

'You can't make an old heifer look like a young cow,' Dido said disparagingly.

Nana's smiled faded and she blinked.

I gave Dido a look, guilt settling in my stomach. I was the one who had called him over to see and brought down his sarcasm on Nana. She got up and shuffled to the bathroom where she scrubbed off the make-up, leaving her face red.

She had been innocently experimenting with something most young girls got the chance to do, and Dido had brought her down again, so when Nana looked up and her face blanched as she looked at my nail polish I was surprised, until I realised Dido was behind me.

Dido approached and took my hand in his. I began to feel wary. Dido wasn't a demonstrative man and I had a portent of danger, but it was too late. He rubbed my fingers, wanting to check if the nail polish would come off. It didn't. He had a cigarette in his mouth and when he dropped my hand he returned to the couch and stubbed out the cigarette in the ashtray.

'*Stara, motika,*' he said, asking Nana to bring him the rod. My eyes widened. Nana slowly hobbled to the kitchen and returned with it.

'Put your hands like this.' Dido joined his fingertips into a point.

'No, no.' I shook my head as I begged.

'Do it,' he commanded.

I looked behind him to Nana, but she kept her eyes on the floor. I lifted my hands up, my fingers joining together. As Dido lifted the rod up to strike, I flinched, quickly hiding my hands behind me.

'Now you're going to get two smacks,' he said.

I was crying as I put my hands back in front of me and closed my eyes. He struck me on the top of my fingers. While Mum had spanked me on the buttocks before, it was the most agonising pain I had ever experienced. As the hard rod struck the tender flesh of my fingertips it felt like they were being flayed.

He hit me once more and then left the house. I ran to my bedroom and closed the door. As I cried my lips formed my mother's name. Although I was angry at her for leaving me here, now that I was in pain all I wanted was the soothing touch of my mum's hands.

My grandparents were collecting rags to sell to a factory and there were a few bags of them in the corner of the bedroom I shared with Haris. I wanted to be anywhere but here. My rage and grief combined and all I could think about was making my grandparents pay. If I was dead they would be sorry.

I got a long piece of cloth and tied it to the stove chimney and knelt. The cloth cut across my neck, making me gasp in pain, but this pain felt good. As I fantasised about my grandfather's guilt and despair when he found my dead body, I felt myself calming and a glow filled me. I held my breath for as long as I could, but soon I needed to breathe in. The cloth was cutting my throat, but I was too chicken to tie it higher and jump to really choke myself. I took off the cloth and threw myself on my bed, and as I stared at the ceiling I wondered what Mum was doing.

POISON PEN

While I was missing my mother in Bosnia, she was experiencing her own tribulations in Australia. Mum felt like she was missing an appendage by leaving us behind, but in Bosnia she had felt like she was suffocating, with the ever-present threat of being admitted to hospital and the horror that awaited her there.

When Mum and Izet returned to Australia, the house she had shared with my father was vacant. Her friends returned the belongings she had asked them to store before she left for Bosnia. The house was furnished and looked as if she had never left, but whenever she walked past our empty bedrooms Mum felt a pang.

Izet began renovating the house. His first job was painting every room and removing the stains of neglect left by years of renters. They settled into the Bosnian social life of exchanging visits with other Bosnians, but Izet was always taciturn and subdued afterwards.

Mum thought it was just because he was a natural introvert and found it hard to socialise, but when her friend Mujo came to visit with his family, she found out what his aversion to Bosnians actually was. Mujo was my dad's best friend and they shared the same uncouth sense of humour. Izet had helped Mujo paint his house the day before.

'I asked him to paint the living room and he painted the

lounge room. What a dill.' Izet's mistake was an easy one to make. In Bosanska Gradiška there wasn't such a thing as a dedicated room just to eat or sit; all spaces were communal and multi-purpose. Mujo was laughing so hard he had turned red. The louder he laughed, the more subdued Izet became. Mujo continued his comedy routine with Izet as the butt of every joke. He laughed about Izet's pronunciation of English when he ordered a sandwich, and about Izet becoming lost when he went to the buy coffee.

'I've had enough.' Izet stood. 'I'm leaving and I won't return until he's gone.'

Mujo found this reaction even funnier, and his peals of laughter chased Izet out.

'Well, I'm going to stay all night until he returns.' Mujo settled into the sofa to wait.

Mum continued talking to Mujo's wife, and she kept glancing at the clock, fretting about where Izet had gone. He knew no one and had nowhere to go. He'd left in such a rush he'd even forgotten his wallet.

'Are you worrying about your beloved?' Mujo teased. 'He's probably lurking outside waiting for me to leave.' He stood and looked through the curtains. 'I'm going to stay all night so he can't come back.'

'Enough,' his wife warned. 'We'll get going.'

After her visitors left Mum cleaned the house, constantly on the alert for Izet's return.

Two hours later she heard the door and rushed into the hallway. 'Where were you?' she asked.

Izet shrugged as he took off his shoes. 'I was walking.'

'I'm sorry about that. Mujo thinks he's funny, but he's not.'

'I'm not visiting any of these people anymore. They are not my friends and I won't waste my time.'

In their time together he had never raised his voice to her, and this was the closest he had ever got. She nodded, knowing not to push. Over the next few months she visited her friends by herself, but it became awkward when it came time for return visits. Izet would always clear out before they came. Some of them would ask if they had done something to offend him, and all she could do was deny it. While she knew that being married would be a challenge, she hadn't realised that their very different personalities would be problematic.

A few weeks after they arrived, Mum received a letter from me. She held the envelope to her chest, feeling as if she was hugging me. We had exchanged letters since she arrived in Australia and she called once a month. Making international phone calls was incredibly expensive. In her first letter she had told me and Haris about how the house was furnished and that our bedrooms were waiting for us when we were ready. I had replied telling her that I missed her and demanding to know when she would return to Bosnia. Mum had had tears in her eyes when she finished reading the letter. Her only hope was that Haris and I would long for Australia and change our minds.

Mum ran into the house and opened the letter. As she read, her excitement turned to horror.

Dear Mum and the pretender who is your husband,
I hope the two of you are having a wonderful time living it up without Haris and me. You chose that pauper over your own flesh

and blood, a man who has nothing and will amount to nothing. If you had gone to a market you would have been able to find a better man by throwing a stone, but you chose this miscreant. I hope that the two of you are enjoying your life, while we live here with nothing. Nana doesn't even have money to buy me new clothes and I have to wear rags. If you can spare some money from your high life maybe you can send some money to Nana so she can buy me some jeans.

Your daughter in name only,
Amra

Mum thought she was going to vomit from the venom dripping from the letter. She re-read it and recognised my grandmother's voice. My grandmother always referred to Izet as a pauper and her constant refrain since Mum had brought him home was that he wasn't good enough for her.

Mum didn't realise that an hour had passed while she lay prostrate on the couch. She had to prepare dinner for Izet, who was out shopping for renovation supplies. She slowly got up, feeling like her whole body was aching after a beating. My words had landed like blows. While she knew intellectually that the letter she'd received was not actually my voice, that my grandmother was using me as a tool of revenge, it was so much more cutting that it was in my handwriting. My grandmother had found the perfect tool to enact her revenge and punish Mum for leaving.

When Izet came home he noticed her mood immediately. 'What's wrong?'

'I received a letter from Amra.' Mum handed him the letter, dreading what would happen when he read it. She watched his face, the way the words slowly worked their way to his soul like a corrosive, taking away all happiness. They spent the rest of the night in subdued silence. Izet let her sit on the couch while he prepared coffee and took care of her.

Every time she went to the letterbox she was filled with dread. She held onto the next letter for fifteen minutes, struggling to find the courage to open it. She opened it only to find a repeat of the venomous tirade. Over the next few months she felt like she was being battered. She missed us, and she felt helpless knowing that my grandmother had free rein to poison us against her.

'I have to go back,' she told Izet.

'I know.'

'You stay here and I'll return with Amra and Haris.'

While she was full of trepidation about being in Bosnia alone, she felt that leaving Izet in Australia tethered her to her old life. With him there, my grandparents could not try to prevent her from leaving again. She prayed that we had missed her and would finally be willing to return home to Australia.

When Mum arrived in Bosnia we attempted to make up for our time apart by staying up all night talking in bed together, once again fighting to take turns lying beside Mum, but things had changed. It had been eighteen months since Mum married Izet and we didn't mesh together. Mum was used to her husband being in bed with her, and Haris and I were used to having our own beds. When Mum asked us to return to Australia to live with her and Izet, we did not put up any resistance. My grandparents' old-fashioned parenting style had well and truly worn thin and I was looking forward to returning to Australia and twenty-first-century attitudes.

Over the next few weeks Mum sent letters to Izet, but when she didn't hear back from him she became concerned. She tried calling him but the phone went unanswered. She called one of her friends to see whether she knew anything.

'He's returning to Bosnia,' her friend told her. 'He should be there by tomorrow.'

Mum hung up the phone, confused. Why hadn't he told her? She waited for him to arrive the next day, but when he didn't show she went to the city. She found him sitting in the bakery where he had once worked. When he saw her his face lit up. He opened his mouth to say something, but she stopped him. She was just relieved that he was there, and that he wanted to be with her. Her whole plan to go back to Australia hinged on them being together.

'Let's go.' She took his hand and led him to her parents' house, where they retreated to her bedroom and closed the door. After months apart, their reunion was hot and passionate. 'Why did you come back?' she asked, as they lay on the fold-out bed together.

'Did you get any of my letters?' Izet asked. Mum shook her head. 'I wrote to you after every letter you sent, but I could see you weren't receiving my letters. I was scared that your parents were turning you against me.'

'They tried, but they failed.' My grandmother had especially tried, spewing a daily tirade whenever Dido was not around, and had used the lack of letters from Izet to prove her point. Mum now realised that Nana must have been destroying them.

They returned to their summer house for the three weeks before our flight to Australia, while my brother and I remained with our grandparents. Mum felt like she was saying goodbye to Bosnia. When she had left the first time as a fifteen-year-old bride she hadn't realised that her life would be in Australia, and that it would become a part of her. Now she knew that Australia was her home and, while she might return to Bosnia for short visits, she would never live there again.

When we got on the aeroplane as a family for the first time and she looked out the window, Mum had a premonition that she would never again see Bosnia. She wondered at this strange sensation. While she knew she would never again live there, she would surely visit. Not for a long time – her bank account was depleted after their numerous jaunts back and forth – but she was sure that she would return sometime in the distant future.

She did not know then that in the years to come the country she grew up in would be ravaged by war, that the borders would be redrawn so the town where she grew up would belong to another country, and that the family she had spent half her life without would be relocated to Australia to live out their old age.

She pushed away her sense of foreboding and let herself feel joy at her new family and the new life that awaited us.

PART III

NERVOUS BREAKDOWNS

I entered the bedroom where my mum was still lying in bed. I had poured myself cereal, then found there was no milk.

'Oh,' Mum said when I told her. She sat up in bed with her hair tousled, blinking sleep out of her green eyes. Izet had left to run errands an hour ago and we were alone. 'Take some money from my purse and go buy it.'

I bit back words of frustration. I missed Nana. During the four years I had lived with my grandparents in Bosnia, I'd find breakfast waiting for me on the table: hot tea, sliced homemade bread, a jar of homemade jam and a stick of butter. In the two weeks I'd been living with Mum again I'd learnt that I would have to fend for myself.

As I rode my bicycle to the milk bar, I enjoyed the sensation of flying. My mood lightened. I looked with curiosity at the yellow and brown brick houses I passed. These were the same streets I'd walked as a young child, but now as a twelve-year-old I looked at them with the eyes of a stranger. This landscape was so different from Bosanska Gradiška. By comparison Melbourne's western suburbs were monochrome and cold. There was concrete everywhere: grey footpaths and asphalt roads, most of the yards lost to concrete driveways.

On my way back home, the plastic shopping bag hanging from my handlebar swung back and forth until its handle tore.

The milk bottle hit the asphalt with a bang, the milk seeping across the black bitumen. I braked abruptly and stared at the mess on the road. I didn't know what to do. I had no money to buy another bottle, as I'd taken only a two-dollar coin from my mother's purse. I began pedalling home.

Fear gripped me the closer I got. I didn't know what Mum would do. If this had happened in Bosnia, my grandfather would have used a *motika* to correct my clumsiness. His preferred method of punishment was beating my fingertips while I held them together. As for my grandmother, she would have chased me away from the house, throwing rocks at my retreating form. Even though I thought she purposely missed with her rock-throwing – surely no one could be that bad – I'd never stuck around to test my theory.

When I arrived home I knocked on the door, because I wanted the option of a quick getaway if Mum got aggro. I had never before been afraid of my mother, but I had become infected with fear.

'Why are you knocking?' Mum asked when she opened the door.

'The milk bottle smashed and it went everywhere on the road.' I was almost in tears.

Mum gave a deep sigh, her lips narrowing with displeasure. 'Here,' she said, handing me a coin.

'Thanks.'

I walked back to my bike, worrying at my lip. Maybe living with Mum was going to be better than living with my grandparents.

Over the following months there were many adjustments as

we learnt to live together as a family. A few nights later I was woken up by strange sounds. I tiptoed out of my bedroom and down the hallway. My brother was standing outside Mum's bedroom, giggling as he listened to the moaning building to a crescendo behind the wooden door. I couldn't believe it: they were having sex while we were in the house.

My brother began mimicking their sounds of passion and I laughed. We waited for a reaction, but it seemed they were so caught up in the thrall of sex that nothing was getting through. My brother kept moaning, getting louder.

'What's that?' Izet asked.

Haris moaned again, loudly. Izet started swearing and we heard the sound of his footsteps. We ran to my bedroom and locked the door, then leaned our backs against it and wedged our feet on the wall opposite.

It took Izet a minute to come after us – he had to get dressed, after all. He pounded on the door. 'I'm going to teach you a lesson,' he shouted.

Haris kept making moaning sounds as our stepfather ranted from the other side. Izet slammed against the door really hard, like he was about to break it. I covered my mouth and stifled my laughter until he returned to their bedroom. Haris and I remained in the same position for the next half an hour. We could hear Izet shouting and Mum's quieter voice as she attempted to placate him.

'You should sleep here,' I told Haris.

'Yeah, we need to put something in the doorway.'

We wedged my bedside drawers behind the door and slept on my bed head to toe. It took us hours to fall asleep because one of us would start giggling and then we'd be off again.

The next morning Izet gave us the silent treatment, shooting dark looks our way.

'That was very rude,' Mum told us after Izet had left for the day.

'It was rude for us to hear your grunting,' I snapped, while Haris ate his cereal.

Mum bit her lip, but didn't say anything further.

A few weeks later I woke up and got ready for school. I had to set my alarm clock and wake up by myself, make my own breakfast and prepare my own school lunch, although there were days when I snuck into Mum and Izet's bedroom and took lunch money from Mum's purse.

I walked to school blearily. I'd stayed up late reading a book. I hadn't been allowed to browse in the library in Bosanska Gradiška; instead, I had to know what book I wanted and then the librarian would find it while I stood by the door waiting. I hadn't read much in Bosnia, apart from what was on the curriculum. When I returned to Australia and discovered libraries I was in heaven, scouting out shelves and shelves of books and taking whatever I wanted. I had a denim book bag made by a friend of the family. It was a large satchel and I'd go to the library and fill it up until it was so heavy that I'd struggle walking to the train station and back home.

I had fallen in love with the world of Mills and Boon romance novels. There were no surprises and no unexpected twists. My life didn't need any more drama: I just wanted simple escapism and respite. After four years in Bosnia, I spoke English with an accent and lagged behind my peers. I discovered that reading Mills and Boons made my vocabulary improve exponentially. I had to read with a dictionary beside me, and while I learnt what the words meant, I didn't always know how to pronounce them. I once used the word 'chasm' in class, and pronounced the *ch* sound. Another time I said 'cynical', a word I knew very well because every romance hero was described as cynical, yet my peers had no idea what it meant. I felt a strange power from being seen as smarter than my peers, but it also left me feeling out of step. Reading became a compulsion and because no one was enforcing a reasonable bedtime, I could stay up all night and frequently did, but then I paid the price at school, my eyes bleary, snoozing on my desk.

The streets were empty of other students, but this wasn't anything new. I was quite often late and was used to arriving after everyone else was already in class, guiltily sneaking up the back and hoping the teacher wouldn't chew me out. It was only when I reached the school and saw the locked gates and the deserted yard, that I realised what had happened. It was a public holiday. In my rush to get to school on time I had forgotten.

I turned back and went home. When I opened the front door and stepped into the hallway, Mum came out from the living room and started at me stupidly. 'Why aren't you at school?'

'Because it's a school holiday,' I snapped, angry. She should be the one who knew about public holidays. I dropped my backpack and entered the living room. The floor was scattered with cushions from the couch. 'What the …'

That's when I noticed Mum was wearing a dressing gown and nothing underneath. My stepfather was sheepishly sitting on the couch, wearing his T-shirt inside out.

'Yuck,' I shouted, and went to the kitchen. I got a slice

of cheese and two pieces of bread. I'd been running late and skipped breakfast. 'You're fucking gross,' I shouted as I rushed past them.

'Well, what do you expect?' Mum picked up the cushions and put them back on the couch. 'This is the only time we can have some fun.'

My brother's bedroom door opened it and he stood in the doorway, rubbing his eyes.

'You didn't even notice he was home,' I shouted, guilt briefly rising up. I'd forgotten to wake him for school. I slammed my bedroom door behind me.

While we were all struggling with the transition from a dysfunctional single-parent family unit to a nuclear family, my mother was the one with the heaviest burden, mediating between us in her roles as mother and wife.

Mum had spent years thinking about returning to Australia. It was a refuge after the hardships she had endured in Bosnia, and at first it seemed as though she had found her little piece of heaven. We didn't have much money, but she had something she hadn't had for a long time: her own space. She was her own boss once again and living in her own home. She was once again maintaining a relationship with my half-sister, her firstborn daughter, Zehra. Zehra had moved to Melbourne and lived a few suburbs away. Izet had enrolled in a tiling course at TAFE.

What Mum hadn't anticipated was the adjustment that we would all have to make as a new family. At first there were nights of laughter. Izet had an affinity for children and he was able to let go and play like he was a child himself. We would play-fight and wrestle.

'Let's see who can beat me,' Izet shouted, holding up a couch cushion. My brother and I quickly followed suit, and a twenty-minute pillow fight ensued, until we were all flushed and exhausted.

At night we would all gather in front of the television to watch a movie together, Haris lying on the floor on his stomach, me next to him, and Mum and Izet on the couch together. We loved Elvis Presley movies and watched every one that was shown on television.

One day Izet ducked out during a commercial break and when he returned he was wearing my black velvet skirt. He sat on the couch, smiling as he waited for my brother and me to notice.

'Oh my God,' Haris shouted. 'He's wearing a skirt.'

I turned around and began laughing. 'I want to take a photo.' I reached for the camera in the TV cabinet drawer.

'No, you won't.' Izet ran back to the bedroom to change.

'Stop him,' I shouted. Haris chased him and wrapped himself around Izet's legs. I ran in with the camera while Mum followed slowly, laughing at the spectacle.

'No, no photos.' Izet tried to take the camera from me.

'Hold him.' I danced away as I pressed the button to turn the camera on.

Izet wrestled with Haris on the bed. Izet fell off the bed and was wedged between the wall and bed, unable to get up as Haris held his legs. I jumped on the bed, snapping a photo of Izet lying on his back, trying to hide himself with his hands.

'Give it back,' Izet shouted.

'Run, run.' My brother and I ran to my bedroom and locked the door.

Izet followed. 'I want that camera.' He banged on the door.

'I'm going to hide it so you can't find it,' I taunted. I hid the camera in the depths of my wardrobe, under multiple layers of clothes, and we waited another commercial before deciding it was safe to return to the living room.

Izet was sitting on the couch with his arm across Mum's shoulders. As we watched the movie my brother and I kept turning around and giggling.

It would take us months to use the twenty-four frames on the film before we took it for processing, and by then we had all forgotten about the photo of Izet in my black velvet skirt. Much hilarity ensued when we had the film developed and for a few years it was in the photo album – until it disappeared, I suspect when my stepfather stealthily removed it.

As we watched television I kept turning to watch the affection between my mother and my stepfather, feeling jealous of their easy affection. I got up and sat on Mum's lap, hugging her with my arms tight around her throat as I pushed Izet away with my legs. I could barely fit on Mum's lap and my sharp bones dug into her thighs.

'Your bum is hurting me.' Mum pushed me away, reinforcing my feeling of rejection.

Soon Izet's Chaplinesque sense of humour, which I had once found so jovial, began to grate on my nerves.

'Did you see the movie *Baldies Are Pulling Their Hair*?' Izet asked in Bosnian, laughing at my confusion. The jokes came constantly, and all of them at my expense. 'Did you see the movie *A Dry Rag at the Bottom of the Sea*?' He continued teasing, while my answers became shorter and my temper more pronounced.

Soon we were asking Mum to referee. 'Tell him to shut up,' I yelled, while Izet demanded that I show him respect.

One day Izet was watching me in profile. 'Look at your nose,' he said. 'People would think you're my daughter.'

My stepfather had a large and prominent nose, a common Bosnian trait, and he'd learnt early in his life that the easiest way to deal with your foibles was to acknowledge them yourself. He didn't understand the horror and pain that his joke caused me.

'I don't have a fucking big honker nose like you,' I shouted as I stood. 'You've got a fucking ugly nose and I'd never be your daughter.' I stormed out, slamming my bedroom door so hard the house shook with its force.

I heard my stepfather shouting that I needed to learn to respect him, which by now had become his constant refrain. He lacked the insight to see that he could not be both our playmate and our parent: to be one, he had to relinquish the other. Mum attempted to mediate, but all I saw was her defending him and therefore condoning his behaviour. Meanwhile, she could not speak honestly to my stepfather about his role in this stalemate because she was very aware that their relationship was tied with a flimsy string she could break with one wrong word.

The pressure of being the peacemaker took its toll and began to affect her mental health, leaving all of us spinning in our individual orbits as we attempted to survive the latest chapter of our fractured family unit.

THE ACCIDENTAL BRIDE

When I was thirteen years old I'd sit on the living room floor watching television after a busy day at school, the room half lit as the sun set. The palm tree in front of our living room window would dance in the wind.

I loved these moments when the day ended and darkness crept into the room like a warm blanket enveloping me in its embrace. The moment when I had to stand up, close the curtains and turn on the light was approaching, but I felt tired and relaxed, and something about the darkened room invited Mum's confidence.

I turned away from the television towards Mum as confessions spilt from her lips. Some of her revelations were horrible truths that a mother should keep from her daughter; others were stories about my family tree that helped me understand who I was.

Listening was a role I had taken on ever since I was a young child. My mute curiosity and unnatural stillness were a balm to the wounded adults in my life. I became their confidante as they poured forth their heartache, sure in the knowledge that their confessions would be lost in a child's short memory. But I never forgot.

I collected stories and stored them in my memory like prayer beads that I grasped onto and revisited, smoothing out the edges over the years until the stories were formed into a prayer necklace, a continuous loop with no beginning or end, until the day I wrote them down.

On this day my mother would tell me the story of the catalyst of her life.

'When I first saw Delil I was disappointed,' Mum told me.

Delil was my mother's first husband.

'Fatima, isn't he dark and handsome?' Jusufa asked with a smile. Jusufa and her husband were friends of my grandparents and had invited Mum to lunch, telling her that Delil, a young man who had gone to Australia seven years before searching for a better life, had returned to Bosnia and would also be in attendance. Mum went, curious to see this strange man who had the village agog with gossip. To their small, impoverished hamlet he was like a rich movie star whose sparkle might rub off on them all.

When they were introduced Mum nodded, her eyes on the ground, too embarrassed to look him in the eye. At fifteen years old she lagged behind her peers, who were already well versed in their physical preference for the opposite sex. While the adults spoke she snuck looks at Delil and evaluated him. She concluded that he wasn't ugly, but neither was he handsome. He was just an ordinary man with a plain face. Working on a tobacco farm under the harsh Australian sun had browned his skin, and the lines on his face were deep crevices, making him look much older than his twenty-eight years – except for his eyes. They were full of gentleness. He caught her glance and smiled.

Jusufa laughed heartily when she intercepted the look. 'Our young buck passes the test.'

Mum's cheeks flushed and she looked away, her anger a hard ball sitting in her mute mouth.

'Ah, Fatima is a modest young woman,' Jusufa said, misinterpreting her anger as embarrassment.

The visit ended soon after and Jusufa's husband escorted Delil out of the house, leaving the women to chat.

'He's a good man,' Jusufa told my mother as they gathered the dishes and took them to the sink. Jusufa pumped water from the hand pump jutting out of the floor and washed the dishes in the flow. 'He will provide for his family and they won't go hungry.'

Even though Mum knew there were no secrets in her hamlet, she still didn't like that everyone knew how poor her family were. Mum was born in Vukovar, a city in Croatia, and their lives had been prosperous. But as my grandfather noticed that his daughters were coming of age and attracting the interest of boys, he decided to return to Bosnia to ensure that my mother and aunt would wed Muslims. My grandparents had to start again, building up their farming land and Dido's predilection for alcohol became more prominent under this strain.

Mum made her excuses and left as soon as she could. The sun was moving across the sky and she still had many chores to perform before nightfall.

The next day she was watching the cows grazing in a nearby pasture. She loved the quiet as she stood outside. There were no shouting voices, no cruel words biting into her thin flesh, no hard blows making her tremble and shake, just the gentle sounds of wind rustling the leaves in the trees, birds tweeting and chirruping, and the soft breeze caressing her bare arms as the sun warmed her inside out.

'Fatima!' She tensed, afraid that it was her father. She looked up and smiled her relief, waving to Jusufa's husband and the young man from Australia.

'We're going to get your father's permission for you to marry Delil.' Jusufa's husband's voice boomed across the field. 'If you don't want us to continue, speak up now, girl.'

Jusufa's husband was waiting for her answer. She didn't know how this had happened – she had only visited to meet Delil, not to meet her husband. Because her survival at home depended on her ability to avoid drawing attention to herself during my grandparents' fights, she had learnt to block out everything and disappear into her imagination. She didn't know what to say, so she did the only thing she knew how: she imagined herself as a brown field mouse, small and almost invisible. They wandered away and she convinced herself that the strange conversation hadn't happened. She attempted to drift back into the moment of blissful nothingness they had interrupted.

When the cows had had their fill, she led them back to the barn and gave them water and hay. She got the milk pail and the stool and milked them. When she entered the house carrying the fresh milk she was hungry and all she could think about was dinner. She cut herself a wedge of bread and thinly spread it with homemade sour cream.

My grandfather was smoking as he sat on the couch and my grandmother was in the kitchen washing the dishes.

Mum sat at the kitchen table and had just taken her first bite when my grandfather spoke. 'I gave my permission for you to marry Delil,' he told her.

Mum started coughing as the bread went down the wrong way.

My grandfather stood to leave the room, but he hesitated in the doorway. 'I wasn't sure whether I should let you get married so young,' he said. 'But this could be your chance to have a life of luxury and ease in Australia and I didn't want to stand in your way.'

Her appetite gone, Mum went to the bedroom she shared with her sister. She sat on the bed and stared at the wall before her. She didn't understand how things had come to this. All she had done was visit a family friend and now she was marrying a stranger. If this had happened to my fiery aunt Nermina she would have been punching walls and shouting her disagreement, and damn the consequences for the family honour, but Mum was not like that.

The next day Jusufa and her husband came to visit with Delil in tow. 'We thought the young people could go out and get to know each other while we finalise the details of the wedding.'

Delil smiled at her as they walked to the town centre. He bought Mum a blue suit to wear to the registrar wedding, which the shop assistant wrapped into a parcel with brown paper. Afterwards they went to the bakery for cake and coffee. Mum was tongue-tied and her answers to Delil's questions were monosyllabic. On the return home she clutched her parcel. They were walking down an unsealed road with paddocks on each side when Delil took her hand. Mum started with surprise.

It was the first time a man had touched her. He stopped, pulling her towards him, and kissed her. She froze at the strange sensation of a bearded face brushing against hers. After a moment she pushed him away, dropping her parcel, and ran home. She hid in her bedroom and remained there until she heard Delil leave. When she entered the living room she found the parcel on the kitchen table.

Two weeks later it was the night of her wedding. My grandmother came into her bedroom holding a battered suitcase and packed her meagre belongings while Mum sat on the bed.

'Mum,' Mum said, her voice trembling. 'I don't want to get married.'

My grandmother's hands stilled mid-motion folding a blouse. 'Well, it's too late now. You already said yes,' she said briskly.

'But I didn't …' Mum began, trying to explain what had happened.

'It's been decided. And at least you had a choice, which is more than most of us can say.' My grandmother turned her back and continued packing.

Mum retreated to the kitchen, where my grandmother had put on a five-litre pot of water to boil. Mum brought in the copper bathtub and placed it in front of the woodstove. She went to the water pump outside and filled a bucket, then returned inside to pour the cold water into the bathtub. After adding the hot water she dipped her hand in and checked the temperature. It was warm. As she lay in the bath, water lapping her body, she smoothed the soap over her pale skin. She knew what would happen tonight. Someone other than her would touch her body. A man would have the right to lay his hands wherever he wanted. She ran her hands over her breasts. He would be able to touch her here. She soaped herself between her legs. And here.

Mum knew what happened between a man and a woman after they were married. Her cousin Džemila had told her about her wedding night. Džemila was a full-figured girl and the first few nights she kept her legs clenched tight, so her husband was forced to consummate their marriage between her thighs. On the third night he managed to wrench her legs apart and Džemila spoke of the grinding pain as he thrust inside her.

Mum ducked her head under the water, holding her breath, until there was pressure in her head and all her thoughts faded. Her chest constricted and dots appeared in front of her eyes. She surged out of the water, panting for breath, and wiped the water from her face. After she got out, she wiped her skin roughly with a towel.

She dressed in her best skirt and her mother's blouse. It hung loosely on her. She had her father's green eyes, brown hair and thin, wiry build; Nermina was more like their mother.

She emptied the bathtub and returned to her bedroom.

'You look terrible,' Nermina said.

Mum looked down, blinking back tears.

'Don't be so sensitive.' Nermina went to stand behind her. She tucked the flower-patterned blouse into the skirt, arranging the pleats so that it looked more fitted. 'There. That's better.'

'Thank you.' Mum smiled.

'Wouldn't want you to embarrass the family,' Nermina said as she left, looking uncomfortable at Mum's emotion.

After she was dressed all there was left to do was wait. My grandmother bustled in the kitchen while Mum sat at the kitchen table and stared out the window. She noticed her mother wiping her eyes, but she wasn't dicing onion.

Delil knocked at the door. Custom demanded that the

father of the bride give a dowry for marriage, but Mum's family weren't in a position to do that. To get around this, the plan was that her betrothed would arrive with his cousin and 'steal her away'. My grandparents made themselves scarce and Delil escorted Mum to the car, a two-door Fiat 500. Delil pushed the front seat forward so Mum could slide into the back, and Delil joined her. Mum felt her breath constrict in her chest as Delil put his arm on the seat behind her, almost hugging her.

At his parents' house the wedding celebration was underway. There was a lamb on a spit, alcohol on the table and a man playing accordion. The guests cheered as Mum got out of the car, and she forced a smile as they congratulated her.

Some time during the night she found herself on the edge of the party. She looked out into the darkness and imagined running across the fields and gardens, reaching the canal and jumping across the water until she reached her parents' house. She'd take off her muddy, ruined shoes to sneak inside and lie down on her bed.

When her parents woke up in the morning they would accept her presence. Her mother would probably give her the silent treatment for a few days and her father would contain his disappointment until he exploded in a drunken rage. But in the end it wasn't the thought of their reaction that stopped her from running away – it was the fact that it would be assumed she'd run because she wasn't a virgin. From that day forward everyone would look at her with a gleam in their eye. Men would leer at her as soon as she was away from the protection of my grandfather; they would make advances, assuming she was good to go. Women would give her suspicious glances, not trusting her to be around their beaus and husbands.

She'd seen this happen to Džemila after her marriage failed and she returned home to her parents. The difference was that her cousin did not meekly accept the scorn and derision. Instead she spat and scratched the men who dared to touch her with the ferocity of a feral cat, profanity spewing from her lips like lava, scorching those who thought her a loose woman.

Mum heard the guests cheering behind her. It was time for the consummation. Delil's mother and sister came and took her to the house, where they left her in the bedroom to wait. Delil entered a few minutes later, rosy-cheeked and smiling cheerfully. They took their clothes off and lay in bed. He kissed her and after a few perfunctory caresses intercourse began. She didn't experience any pleasure, but after the first thrust she didn't feel any pain either. Soon he was finished and they lay side by side and fell asleep. He woke her again and by the third time she was more annoyed by the loss of sleep than his lustful attention.

She awoke in the morning to find a heavy arm across her chest. She turned to look at her new husband sleeping beside her. Mum had expected that she would feel different – she was a woman now, after all – but apart from a faint throbbing between her legs, she was the same person who had gone to sleep last night. She had always known that she would be married, and while she had expected it to be a few years off yet, it was not unknown for a girl of her age to be married or even become a mother.

After they were dressed his mother came into the bedroom and took the sheet. She hung it on the clothes line for everyone to view the bloodstain proving Mum's chastity, an old-fashioned custom that was expected of all new brides.

The next day my mother and Delil went into town and got married legally at the registry office wearing the blue suit he had bought her, her parents in attendance to provide their signatures allowing their fifteen-year-old daughter to wed a man she'd met fifteen days before.

As I looked out the living room window at the palm tree, a maelstrom of emotion swirled through me. 'How could you do it?' I asked. 'How could you marry a stranger?'

'They were different times,' Mum told me. 'Most couples barely knew each other because a woman was not allowed to be alone with a man.'

Mum lay back on the couch, as if the telling had exhausted her, and I watched her as she dozed. I was seeing her differently. I had judged her for so long for the way her choices had negatively affected my life, but now I was getting a glimmer that she was as much a victim of circumstance as I was.

BURGEONING BEAUTY

My mother's friend Aida approached Mum and hugged her hard. 'Congratulations!' She looked down at Mum's stomach. 'When is the baby due?'

Mum looked like she'd been slapped and blinked back tears. 'I'm not pregnant.'

Before she went to Bosnia, Mum used to do sit-ups every night after my brother and I went to bed, and she was always careful with her portions. While we had been living with my grandparents it was unseemly for Mum to exercise in front of my grandfather, nor did she have the time. Slowly her weight had crept up and now her stomach had formed into a hard ball that resembled a five-month pregnancy. She was wearing cheap fleece tracksuit pants that made her look frumpy and middle-aged.

'And look at your Amra.' Aida turned to me and looked me up and down. 'You're a proper woman now.'

I had entered adolescence, my body blossoming. I got pains in my chest as my breasts grew and they were perfectly round and perched on my chest like two grapefruit halves. The navy cord pants of my school uniform became obscenely tight as my hips developed. I had to lie down and fight with the zipper in order to tug them on, and the seams left angry red welts on my flesh by the end of the day.

'You must have all the boys looking at you.'

I nodded shyly. I'd noticed the boys scanning the way the navy cord gripped my buttocks and thighs, and their scrutiny had inspired my vanity. Every morning I put on Ponds face cream, a thick, oily moisturiser that made my skin shine for hours until it was absorbed, leaving me glowing. I used to bathe in oil water so that my whole body was moisturised. I had thin eyelashes and read that castor oil would thicken them, so I washed out an old mascara tube and filled it with castor oil. Every night before I went to bed I brushed castor oil onto my eyelashes. When I woke during the night to go to the toilet, the castor oil had seeped into my eyes and made it hard to see. The bathroom door was right next to my bedroom so I was able stumble to the bathroom and back by touch.

Being witness to my transformation made my mother nostalgic for her own days of beauty. Her stories featured her as the femme fatale and everyone else was a supporting actor.

'Your father was as handsome as a movie star,' she told me after Aida left. She knew I couldn't resist a good story; as she expected, I turned down the television and turned towards her, my eyes wide with curiosity.

'When we entered a room together, all eyes were on us,' Mum said, and I shivered, remembering the sensation of the boys at school bathing me with admiration. 'When I was young,' Mum began, 'all the men wanted me. One night your father took me to a *Zabava* and there was a famous folk singer from Bosnia on the stage. I'd dyed my hair platinum blonde, and as he performed his favourite song about a blonde woman, he came to our table and serenaded me.' Mum sighed heavily, caught up in the memory.

I imagined how Mum must have felt as the handsome singer's eyes drank her in, loving the sensation of my father, beside her, being sidelined for once. My father had thought nothing of flirting with pretty women in front of Mum, and she had had to pretend that she didn't mind. Now finally he was on the receiving end.

Once my parents had stopped at a red traffic light and a motorbike rider had pulled up next to them, long, flowing hair cascading out from the helmet. My father had rolled down the window, leaning his elbow out of the car. 'Hello, love,' he'd called out, a charming smile on his lips.

The motorbike rider turned a bearded face towards him. My father quickly ducked back into the car, winding up the window. When the light turned red he throttled the gas, screeching away, while my mother turned her head, not daring to laugh out loud.

As the folk singer finished his song, he held my mother's hand to his lips and kissed it before going back on stage. 'Your father was so jealous. He didn't allow me to dye my hair after that.'

I sighed, imagining the romance of it all.

After Aida's visit Mum sought to reclaim her waistline. When I woke up in the morning, the smell of bleach would punch me in the face. Mum was exercising in front of the television, doing sit-ups, push-ups and leg lifts. She'd spent the night cleaning the walls with a tea towel and a bucket of warm bleach water, wiping them down one strip at a time, removing the yellow patina left by cigarette smoke. Her hands were wrinkled and pruned from the water, and dry from the bleach. When Mum finally went to bed in the early hours of the morning she would toss and turn, feeling restless and jittery. It was as if there were ants crawling on her skin, and as soon as she scratched one itch, another would start in a different part of her body. She would fall asleep for a few hours, only to wake up at dawn to exercise.

As my stepfather twigged to the fact that Mum was going off the rails, he'd try to convince her to take her medication. She avoided the topic. If he pressed she would put a pill in her mouth, but there were times I would go to the bathroom and find tablet residue around the sink.

When we left for school one day she got in the car.

Izet ran out of the house. 'Where are you going?'

'To the shopping centre.' Mum turned on the ignition.

'I don't think that's a good idea.' Izet leaned down and peered in the side window. 'You haven't slept all night. Why don't you come inside and have a rest, and then you can go?'

'No, I need to go shopping.' Mum pressed her foot to the pedal and the car shot out of the driveway.

A driver coming down the street hit the brakes, just barely missing her boot.

'Sorry.' Mum raised her hand quickly in apology.

When Mum arrived at the shopping centre she went to Copperart. Dazzled by the shiny brass furniture and glass tabletops, she bought a telephone stand, a television table and a coffee table.

'How much money did you spend?' Izet asked when she came home with the boxes.

'Not much.' She didn't know the amount. She had just fluttered from item to item, buying whatever she wanted.

'How are we going to pay the bills?' Izet asked. 'You can't spend money like this. We don't have any more.'

'It's my money.' Mum ripped open a box. 'I can do what I like with it.'

Izet left the house and Mum spent the afternoon in a frenzy, opening boxes and assembling furniture. After she had arranged everything to her satisfaction she scoured her linen cupboard and found her crocheted doilies, which she artfully arranged on the glass-topped coffee table and lamp stands.

When I came home from school Mum held out her arms to encompass the new living room and asked, 'What do you think?'

'It's very shiny.' I was revolted by the cheap glass and brass furniture. I sat on the couch and turned on the television. 'What's for dinner?'

'I haven't had a chance to cook,' Mum said. 'I was too busy shopping. We can get takeaway.'

'We can?' Takeaway was almost taboo in our household. My mother had learnt to stretch her pension to cover all the necessities of living, helped by the fact that we had no mortgage because my father's life insurance had paid off the house. The only version of takeaway pizza we had eaten was Mum's, when she used a Turkish bread as a base and threw on toppings she'd bought from the deli.

'Sure,' Mum said. 'What do you want?'

'We're getting takeaway,' I shouted when Haris walked in the front door from school.

'We are?' Haris said. 'But you always say we don't have money.' Haris took in the living room furniture and his eyes widened with delight. 'Wow, shiny.'

'We do now. Here.' Mum took out a note and handed it to me. 'Go get yourselves pizza.'

There was a pizza shop around the corner and Haris and I raced each other to the door.

When we returned we ate the pizza, while Mum watched. Izet tried to get her to take her medication, but she argued with him.

'I think tomorrow we need to see Dr Keddy,' Izet said.

'I can't.' Mum started doing stretches. 'I need to start racing tomorrow. I need to practise so I can race Evelyn Ashford in the Olympics.'

'Fatima, you're not going to race anyone. You need help. You're getting sick.'

'No, I'm not. You're just trying to stop me from racing.' Mum tore herself out of his arms and went outside, where she started running around the backyard.

Haris scrunched closer to Izet on the couch and I retreated to my bedroom. At this point my coping mechanism was to disappear into a Mills and Boon novel, while my brother would cling tighter to my stepfather.

With Mum out of earshot Izet made a phone call. An hour later there was a knock on the door. I peered out of my bedroom and saw Izet let in three people, one of them Vera, my mother's mental health case manager. I followed them to the living room.

'Good evening, Fatima,' Vera said. 'Izet told me you're having some trouble.'

Vera was a part of the Crisis Assessment and Treatment team and oversaw Mum's medical care in an attempt to minimise her hospital admissions. She had been allocated to Mum because they spoke the same language, although they were of different ethnicities. The CAT team were there to assess whether Mum needed to be hospitalised or could be treated at home.

Mum shot Izet a dark look. 'I'm not having any trouble. I'm feeling the best I have in the world. I was just training for my big race.'

'Yes, your husband was just telling us about that.' Vera smiled and started asking Mum questions. After a few minutes she concluded: 'We think you should come to the hospital for a little while to be treated. Why don't you pack a few things?'

As I watched Mum following the CATT team out to the car, telling them about her big race, I felt a sense of déjà vu. This was a scene I had witnessed many times as a child, but this time would be different. When Mum went to hospital before she married Izet, life, as Haris and I knew it, would stop. At least now we got to go to the same school, hang out with our friends, stay in the same house. Life continued as normal, just quieter.

RITES OF PASSAGE

When I woke my head was throbbing, and my back and pelvis muscles ached. I lolled on the couch trying to watch *Rage*, feeling uncomfortable. During a commercial break I went to the toilet and saw blood on my underwear. I had only found out about periods when I started high school, from my girlfriends. My grandparents had kept me sheltered while I lived with them. Even though I knew what a period was, I'd somehow never realised that I would be afflicted with them.

I stuffed toilet paper into my underwear then yanked the phone into my bedroom, stretching the cord to its limit, and closed the door. The phone rang out once. 'Oh God, please be home,' I begged as I dialled again.

'What?' Zehra's voice finally came on. She sounded half-asleep and belligerent. She had moved to Melbourne six months before and was living in a share house in St Albans.

'It's Amra,' I whispered.

'Who?'

I repeated my name again, louder.

'Why are you calling so early?' Zehra moaned.

'I got my period,' I whispered, aware of my stepfather in the living room.

'So? Hang on, is this your first period?'

'Yes,' I said. 'I don't know what to do. Mum is in hospital and I can't talk to Izet.'

'Didn't mum buy you pads?'

'No.' My tears gathered. 'I put in some toilet paper, but I don't know how long it's going to work.'

'Okay, I'm coming over.'

I hung up the phone and waited at the front of the house. A few minutes later I saw a red Commodore ute pull up and Zehra got out.

'Here, take these,' she said, handing me a plastic bag with pads. 'This should last you a couple of days and if you need any more you can call me. Make sure you change them frequently.'

The guy in the car beeped the horn.

'Gotta go. I'll come by tomorrow. We'll talk then.' Zehra waved as she got back in the car.

The driver did a screeching burnout as they disappeared around the corner. I returned home, put a pad between my legs and went to bed. The throbbing in my back had increased and now cramping had started in my abdomen. When I woke, Mum had come home for a weekend stay and was eating breakfast in the kitchen. The medication was flattening her mood and I could see she was lethargic.

'You're being lazy today,' she snapped as soon as she noticed me. 'The least you can do is wash the dishes.' She pointed at the full sink.

I avoided housework at the best of times and this didn't change while Mum was in hospital. Izet picked up the slack, but still there would be some cleaning waiting for Mum whenever she was home for the weekend.

But now at least I had a genuine reason for my slackness.

I felt heavy and defeated by the force of what was happening to my body, and worn down by pain. 'I got my period,' I whispered.

'Oh.' Mum went silent for a moment. 'Do you need pads?'

'No, I got some from Zehra.' I enjoyed seeing the consternation on her face. She had failed to prepare me for this rite of passage. 'I need you to buy more.'

'I'll tell Izet to add it to his list,' Mum said. My stepfather was the one who did the grocery shopping while Mum was in hospital.

'What? No, I don't want him to buy them for me.'

Mum didn't say anything.

'Just give me money and I'll do it myself,' I said.

She handed me a note.

I was angry with her for ages, angry that she didn't prepare me for this brutal transition from girl to woman, but then I heard the story of her becoming a mother and my anger faded.

In December 1969, three months after her wedding, Mum stepped out of the aeroplane with her first husband, Delil, squinting as the harsh Australian sun felt like it could peel away layers of her skin. She was three months pregnant and suspected she had conceived on her wedding night. She noticed the faded blackness of the tarmac, the muted colours of the buildings, the way that the sun glinted off the aeroplanes and stabbed her cornea.

Delil's brother, Tarik, and his friend greeted them at the gate. The friend had been borrowing Delil's car; he'd returned it so that Delil could drive his new bride home. Mum looked on in wonder: only the wealthiest people in Bosnia had a vehicle.

Mum stared out the window, watching the landscape that was so different to her home. Bosnian forests were lush and green, with tall, brown tree trunks and wide canopies. Here the trees were more like bushes, the tree canopies sparse, the grass yellow and bleached by the harsh summer sun.

'Here we are.' Delil nodded out the window three hours later. 'This is Myrtleford.'

She looked at the poplars that stood tall like sentries guarding a treasure, which lined the road leading into town. Mum saw a sign with the number 2,741 on it.

'What does that mean?' she asked.

'That is stating the number of people that live here.'

'What a strange custom? My-tle …' Mum tried pronouncing the name, but the stress syllables were opposite to Bosnian pronunciation.

'Myrtleford. It was named after the local creek which had myrtle trees growing on its banks.'

It was the pastoralists who had named it in 1837. The town had a close-knit community and the biggest crime wave was a trio of youths stealing money from milk bottles in residents' front yards, left out for the morning milk delivery.

In the town centre there were one-storey structures with signs that Mum couldn't read. Within a few minutes they'd passed through the town, and trees and pastures once again lined the road.

Fifteen minutes later Delil parked in front of a weather-beaten fibro house that he shared with his brother. The owner-grower leased the house to a perpetual stream of share-crop farmers, like Delil and Tarik. During his seven years in Australia Delil had become adept at managing the household chores, and the faded linoleum and creaking floorboards were clean, but nothing could disguise the forlorn house's air of neglect from years of temporary tenants seeking shelter within its walls.

While Mum was slightly disappointed – she had been told that people in Australia lived like royalty and she had expected something much grander – the house was still more spacious than her parents' home in Bosnia. There were three bedrooms and an open-plan kitchen and living room.

Mum barely slept that night as her body acclimatised to the time difference. At five in the morning Delil woke her and her first day as a tobacco farmer's wife began. She helped him make sandwiches for their field workers and she cooked goulash for their lunch, and then they went out to the fields.

Life was dictated by the seasons of the harvest. In August Mum helped plant seedbeds, which were covered overnight with sheets of plastic. These seeds were nurtured tenderly, and during cold weather Delil and the other men stayed up all night lighting fires to keep the seedlings warm so they wouldn't be killed by frost. In October the seedlings were ready to be planted into the paddocks. This process was partially mechanised: Mum and Delil would work on a tractor-drawn planter. The planter had large metal discs that cut through the earth to create furrows, a mechanised wheel that inserted the seedlings, and side wings that pushed the earth down around the plants.

When Mum arrived the plants were growing and her daily chore was weeding the garden beds using a hoe and 'topping' the plants to remove the flower while it was in bud, to increase the overall yield per hectare. New shoots called suckers would appear on the plants, which had to be manually broken off and discarded.

Each row was one kilometre long and she was bent over as she dug from one end to the other, while the sun rose higher in the sky, burning her fair skin and bathing her in sweat. She was used to hard work, having grown up on a farm, but this was a new reality. In Bosnia she had helped her parents farm their land so they could grow their own produce. In Australia she was a labourer working in the paddock.

At lunchtime she got a reprieve when she went inside to serve lunch. She'd been working for five hours straight, her only breaks used to drink water and use the toilet. She was tired, sweaty and sore.

After lunch she walked to the paddock and picked up her hoe. Mum stood swaying like a blade of grass in the breeze as she looked at the paddock before her. It seemed to stretch into infinity. She went to the end of the row and began digging. Her hands were sore with calluses and after her break she felt like she was holding fire as the wood rubbed against her tender palm.

That night she went to bed tired and aching, her back muscles throbbing in pain from the hard toil. The days passed, and months. Soon she was used to waking up at 5 a.m. and working in the paddock all day, stopping only to prepare meals and clean the house. Her pregnancy advanced and her stomach grew, but there were no concessions. It was all hands on deck whatever the weather.

Harvest began in February, when she was five months pregnant. Leaves ripened from the bottom of the plant to the top, and the men picked the ripe leaves six times until the plant had been completely harvested. The leaves were transported to the kilns. The women worked in a shed, tying leaves into bunches and hanging them to dry, while the kiln fire burnt all day. She worked in the shed with the Italian women and Besima who was her new sister-in-law. Tarik had married a few months before and they had moved out to their own house nearby. When the leaves were dry the women classified them into bales, ready for sale to tobacco companies.

The work in the shed was still hard, like working in an oven – Mum sometimes felt like she was a chicken basting slowly in her own juices – yet she was grateful not to be bent over digging all day. Her discomfort advanced along with her pregnancy, but there was no respite from work and she had learnt to do what was expected from her.

Although it was midwinter, Mum was soaked with sweat from standing in the hot shed all day. At nine months pregnant the baby was pressing heavily on her bladder and she had to go to the toilet frequently. She had just finished urinating and had pulled up her panties when she felt water rushing down her thighs with the force of a cow's gushing stream. She walked out of the toilet, embarrassed and shaken.

Isabella, the farm owner's wife, was waiting outside and asked, 'What's wrong?'

'I peed myself.'

Isabella looked down at her wet legs and dress. 'Your waters just broke,' she told her. 'You're going into labour.'

Mum looked down at the rivulets of fluid on her legs. Apprehensive, she felt like she was floating above her body like a bird. Although she had grown up on a farm, she was ignorant of the mechanics of birthing. My grandparents did not believe that young girls should know such things and had sent her away whenever the topic was discussed, in order to shield her. So while she knew that a baby came out of the vagina, she did not know much else. Isabella led her home, where Mum got changed and packed a few things before Delil took her to hospital. The agony of childbirth would be a crucible, shaping the life of suffering that awaited her.

After they arrived at the hospital Delil signed her in and completed the paperwork. A nurse came and led Mum down the corridor. She turned to her left, but Delil was no longer there. She looked over her shoulder and saw him walking out of the hospital.

'Delil,' she called, but he didn't stop.

The nurse said something and Mum tried to understand what she was saying. Panic was sweeping over her in waves, like a tsunami destroying all in its wake. Mum didn't understand English. In the six months she'd been in Australia she had mostly interacted with Bosnians: Tarik, Besima and another family that lived nearby. The Italian owners spoke their own mother tongue to each other, so she hadn't had the opportunity to learn much English and what little she did know was broken and basic.

She entered the labour room and pain was soon sweeping over her in punishing waves. Just when she'd caught her breath, another wave would come. She felt as if her body was being cleaved in two by a sadistic woodchopper's axe. The nurses and doctors spoke to each other. She tried to understand what they were saying, but the words were too rapid. The one thing she could understand was the worry that coloured the doctor's face after he examined her.

Hours passed in a blur of pain and exhaustion. She retreated somewhere deep inside herself, where everything was dark. She could still hear the nurses and the doctors, she could faintly hear the grunts of pain that slipped out of her, and yet her consciousness split. There was the girl who was lying on the table, her body fighting a war to expel the baby that inhabited her, and there was the girl who existed before she'd met Delil. The girl who had stood in the meadow, feeling the soft breeze caressing her bare arms and the sun on her skin.

Her reprieve came when she felt the pressure of a scalpel slicing her perineum. She would learn later that after a twelve-hour labour her doctor, Dr Smith, had performed an episiotomy, deciding that the baby was not going to come out on its own. There was a wrenching motion as the baby was expelled, as if she were a champagne cork. She heard the baby crying and wept with relief.

Mum told me that she'd wanted to name her firstborn Amra, after her favourite cousin, but the custom was that my sister had to be named after her maternal grandmother. Mum was in hospital for seven days, which was mandatory for new mothers at the time. Delil took her home and the next day she was back in the shed classifying tobacco while the baby remained in her cot in the house. Sometimes when Mum returned to the house to feed the baby she found her lobster red from crying. Mum mechanically fed and burped her, changed her nappy and returned her to the cot, her hands on autopilot.

My mother told me she didn't know she had to talk or interact with a baby, and even if she had known she wouldn't have had the time. She had to get back out onto the farm.

She was full of energy and verve. Her sleep was regularly interrupted for night feeds and she was working hard during the day, yet she was unable to be still. Even when she lay in bed to sleep her body twitched and it felt like ants were crawling on her, tickling her, and in the morning her skin would be red with scratch marks.

Mum was working in the shed when everyone began drifting away for smoko. Since coming home she'd been feeling disconnected and lonely, like a balloon floating into the clouds, her life on the farm a stark contrast to the bevy of social activity she'd been exposed to in the hospital.

Isabella sat down next to Mum. 'I need a coffee hit.' She sighed as she fanned her face with her hand.

'You come my house for coffee?' Mum asked.

Isabella smiled. 'I'd love to. I'd love to see your beautiful daughter.'

'She beautiful like Mum,' Mum said as they walked. 'People say I'm like movie star.' They had reached her house and Mum opened the flyscreen for Isabella.

As they walked in they could hear Zehra grizzling. Mum picked up her daughter and changed her nappy. After breastfeeding her, Mum started preparing coffee while Isabella held the baby against her shoulder and rubbed her back to burp her.

'I going to be movie star,' Mum said as she prepared the coffee cups. 'I go on *New Faces*.' *New Faces* was an Australian talent show.

'You're going on *New Faces*?' Isabella asked, sceptical.

'Yes, yes. Frankie say I win.'

'Frankie who?' Isabella asked.

'You know, man on show.'

'You mean Frank Wilson?'

'Yes, Frankie say I look like movie star.' Mum pointed to the television. 'He talk to me and say I talented.' Mum started singing, stringing together a mixture of English and Bosnian words. As she talked about her grandiose dreams of stardom, her speech became slurred and Isabella had to keep repeating back what she was saying, trying to understand her. Isabella left after they'd had coffee and avoided Mum for the rest of the work day.

That night Delil came home from work looking concerned. 'What did you say to Isabella?' he demanded.

'Nothing. We talked about Frankie.' As Mum explained her dreams, Delil sat down on a kitchen chair and stared at the floor.

The next day he took Mum to see Dr Smith, who had already formed a suspicion about her malady. He diagnosed puerperal psychosis. It is a type of postpartum depression that affects one or two out of every 1000 women who give birth, and it often leads to bipolar disorder later in life. Dr Smith referred her to a psychiatrist and Delil told her he was taking her to see a doctor in Melbourne.

Tarik and Besima stood on the porch, her sister-in-law holding the baby in her arms.

Everything felt distant and strange, as if a parasitic creature had taken control of her body. When they hit traffic Mum said, 'You'd better drive faster or I'm going to take over.'

'You don't have a licence,' he replied, looking at her strangely.

'I don't need one. I can do it.'

When they arrived at the hospital in Melbourne Delil went to speak to the receptionist.

Mum walked down the corridor while she waited. She peered into an open room and saw an old woman lying in bed, shaking her legs in the air. The woman had no underwear.

Mum flushed and looked away. *Why am I here with this whore?* she wondered.

When she returned to reception she saw Delil walking out of the hospital. She followed and called his name, but he got in the car and slammed the door, driving away with a screech of tyres.

A nurse approached her. 'Let's go, Fatima?' she said, taking her arm.

'Where am I?' Mum asked in Bosnian. 'Why am I here?'

The nurse answered, but Mum could make no sense of what she was saying. She held her chest as she walked. It had been hours since she'd fed her baby and her nipples tingled as if a phantom child was latched on and suckling, leaving a milk discharge on her blouse as she leaked.

My mother was subjected to electric shock treatment, a routine treatment for mental illness at the time. The only images I had of electric shock treatment were from the movie *One Flew Over the Cuckoo's Nest*, where Jack Nicholson's character is strapped onto a gurney, a plastic plug is placed in his mouth, and his body convulses as electricity jolts through his body.

My mother didn't remember much about her treatment. She remembered being woken up three times a week by a nurse standing at the foot of her bed. The nurse would escort her to the treatment room, where she would be sedated and have a rubber block inserted in her mouth so she wouldn't bite her tongue. She would wake up hours later in her hospital bed, in agonising hunger because she'd missed breakfast, watching the clock as she waited for the lunchtime food tray.

What she did remember was the feeling of abandonment because her husband had left her without explaining why. As she told me this story, a tear trickled down her cheek. Even though twenty years had passed, it was as if she was telling me a story about something that had happened the day before.

Four months after she was admitted, Mum was released. While her psychosis was cured, she was forever vulnerable to her brain's chemical imbalance.

SUITCASE

'There is one simple thing you can do to help yourself,' said the psychologist running the information session at Mum's hospital. 'You can pack a suitcase and leave it in your bedroom when you feel symptoms taking hold. This way if you're admitted into hospital in a hurry, you will have what you need.'

Mum lifted her head. She'd been in hospital for three days. The medication had flattened her and brought her out of the delusional state; her manic energy and verve were gone, leaving her lethargic and depressed. When we visited we would find her in bed. She would struggle to get up, walking to the visiting room with bowed shoulders, looking like she was carrying baskets of rocks on her shoulders.

Mum tuned out as the psychologist spoke and instead pictured her brown suitcase. Delil had bought it for her before they travelled to Australia. The suitcase was tanned leather and had a fibreboard and plywood frame that protected her belongings in transit. The base had domed brass feet to protect it from the ground. On the top were shiny nickel-plated hasp locks that opened with a key, so the dangly hasp was released with a loud snap. The suitcase was old and weary. It had travelled with her from house to house, and country to country.

When she wasn't using the suitcase it remained on top of her wardrobe; she threw all her important documents in it, leaving them in a jumbled mess that she would transfer to a box when she needed to use it. The suitcase was like an old friend that had witnessed her life over more than twenty years. She felt a calm descend over her. Now she had a plan for her illness and would be sure to prepare herself.

Mum was released home three weeks later. Her symptoms had subsided but she struggled to get out of bed and could only manage a few hours of housework before having to lie down on the couch. She attempted to go grocery shopping, but had to turn back after experiencing panic attacks. Soon she gave up driving completely. Izet took over the grocery shopping and ferried her to and from doctor's appointments.

Izet's homesickness persisted. My brother had accepted Izet as Dad, even before he had married Mum, but I wasn't given to trust. I had seen too many of Mum's former beaus pass through and expected Izet to do the same. Once we moved to Australia together I contemplated accepting him as my father, and had even been on the verge of calling him Dad, but then his rants began and my trust evaporated.

Any negative interaction with people outside our family would confirm to him that this was a 'shit country' and he would talk about going 'home' to Bosnia. But the Bosnia he talked about was the country of his youth and didn't exist anymore. His stories were about his golden childhood being outdoors – swimming in the Sava River, going fishing and bringing food home. This wasn't the Bosnia of his adulthood.

Unbeknown to us, Mum's patience was also wearing thin. When her illness was dormant Mum was a gentle soul. She didn't swear, and the only faux profanity she would lob at my brother and me was *jebem ti robiju*, which translated to 'fuck the prison'. She was scared of shouting and if one of us raised our voice she would back down, leaving us to rage while she listened in silence, and then played peacemaker when calm finally returned. She used this same technique to manage my stepfather's ranting. But when she had a manic episode her inhibitions were down and all the things she thought but never gave air to exploded from her in a violent burst that left everyone stunned.

The tensions in the household worked like a pressure cooker. Once again Mum began suffering from insomnia, before progressing to full-blown mania.

'*Stara*, I think we need to go to the hospital,' Izet said.

Mum remembered her brown suitcase and went to the bedroom. She tipped out the paperwork and threw the suitcase on the floor. She had opened the wardrobe when Izet came in.

'I've just called Vera. Why don't you come to the couch and wait for her?' He took Mum's arm and tried to lead her back to the living room.

'I'm busy.' Mum shook him off.

'Stop it. You need to calm down.' Izet voice cracked under the strain.

'You stop it. You're the reason I'm sick. If it wasn't for you, I would be fine.'

Izet backed up and stood in the doorway, watching her in shock. This was the first time Mum had said anything that could be construed as criticism of him.

'I want you gone,' Mum shouted.

'Please, *Stara*,' he pleaded, his hands in the air in surrender.

'I've had enough of you. You keep saying you hate Australia and you hate living here, so go.'

Izet crumpled like a broken man.

'Here, I'll help you.' She reached into the wardrobe and scooped out Izet's clothes, tossing them into the open suitcase. When it took too long she started throwing his clothes out the window, his tracksuit pants, T-shirts and tops littering the front lawn like an abstract sculpture.

'Mum, maybe you should calm down.' I approached her. While I had wanted Mum to take my side – and I had even secretly wanted her to confront Izet about his desire to leave – now that it was happening I was terrified he would actually walk out.

'You said you want him gone too,' Mum said. 'Now I'm sending him away. I want him out of my life.'

Izet returned to the living room and Mum pursued him, harsh words spewing from her lips. All the things she had kept to herself as she listened to his constant negativity and criticisms. Things that she had hidden in the recesses of her mind and tried to pretend that she'd never thought –now they'd become bullets aimed straight for her Izet's heart. Why did she ever think that she needed him? She was strong. She didn't need a man. She didn't need anyone in her life. She had spent so many years without him. She could do it again. He could leave any time and return back to the pauper's existence she had saved him from. As she ranted Izet collapsed on the couch and cried in gulping sobs, her words spinning like a typhoon around him.

Eventually she calmed down, the CATT team came and admitted her to the hospital, and the cycle of recovery, rehabilitation and reconciliation began again. I thought that Izet would leave – after all, their marriage had begun based on a mutual need– but I had underestimated their mutual dependence. While Mum needed Izet as a crutch for her mental illness, Izet needed her just as much. He had nothing to return to: his family had been marked during World War II and the stain had pervaded the family tree. His siblings had thrived by leaving their hometown, and this was Izet's only escape.

During World War II Izet's parents were having dinner when there was a knock on the door. They looked at each other with concern. Bosanska Gradiška was on the banks of the River Sava, which was the border between Croatia and Bosnia, a precarious geographic location as the axis of power was constantly shifting. When the Partizans, who fought with the Allies against Germany, would break the front line and search for men to conscript, the women would hide them under a quilt and sit on them, pretending to drink coffee and gossip. At other times the Ustaše, the Black Shirts – members of the Croatian fascist and ultranationalist movement who believed in a racially pure Croatia and weren't afraid to use genocide to achieve their dream – would search for Partizans or their sympathisers to interrogate.

Izet's father, Murat, opened the door and three Black Shirts pushed in, filling the small house with their menacing presence. 'We need you to come with us,' the leader said to Murat.

'Why?' Murat asked.

'We need people with your skills,' the leader said. 'We need shoemakers for our factory in Zagreb.'

Zagreb was the capital of Croatia and the centre of the revolution. Izet's mother, Esma, opened her mouth to speak, but Murat shook his head and she swallowed her objection.

Murat looked down with resignation, while Esma wiped her tears. 'Let me finish my dinner,' Murat said.

The leader took out his gun and pointed it at Murat. 'Now,' he demanded, his eyes hard and flat.

Murat lifted his hands in surrender, while Esma gathered their children around her, her sobs breaking through as she watched her husband being led away. At this time Murat and Esma had been married for three years and had two children. Murat made a move towards his family, wanting to hug them goodbye, but the Black Shirts bundled him out the front door and away.

He was gone for four years, toiling in a factory, making shoes for Ustaše soldiers, while his wife and children struggled to survive the war without him. Esma went back to live with her parents.

It seemed like a miracle when Murat returned to Bosanska Gradiška. He dug up the gold coins he had hidden in the backyard and used them to buy shoemaking tools. He opened a shop in town. Two months later two men entered his shop, the logos sewn on their shirts identifying them as Partizans. They introduced themselves as Tomo and Ivo.

'How can I help you gentleman?' Murat asked, painfully aware that they had brought no shoes for repair.

'This is a nice shop,' Tomo said, while Ivo examined everything. The shop was a hole in the wall with just enough space for Murat to undertake his craft.

'Thank you,' he said.

'Did you enjoy your time in Zagreb?' Tomo asked.

'No, I didn't,' Murat said. 'The Ustaše conscripted me.'

'Did they?' Ivo asked, a smirk on his face. He leaned over

the counter and picked up the welting awl that Murat used to poke holes in leather.

'You know that capitalism is not allowed in a communist society, Comrade,' Tomo said.

'I'm providing a service,' Murat said. 'People need their shoes repaired.'

'Yes, but they don't need them repaired by a collaborator. We need to take your tools.'

Ivo came behind the counter and began throwing Murat's tools into a box.

'Don't,' Murat implored, reaching out to stop him. His finely crafted shoemaking tools were from Germany and he had scrimped and saved for years to buy them. He would never be able to replace them all. 'I won't be able to make a living.'

'That's not our problem, Comrade,' Tomo said, and the two of them left.

'Why are you home early?' Esma asked him when he returned home.

'It's all gone.' Murat had sat for what seemed like hours in the shop. Finally he had turned off the light and locked the door behind him, knowing it was the end of his dream.

'What's gone?' Esma asked.

'The Partizans took my tools.' He ripped off his shirt and threw it on the ground. 'They say I was an Ustaše collaborator.'

'But that's not true.'

'They don't care.'

'God, what will happen to us?' Esma sat on the couch looking at her husband with despair.

A month later Murat was rounded up with other

collaborators. They were held as prisoners in the basement of a local cafe. Murat knew that he would be executed or put in prison – either way his life was over.

'Murat, is that you?' a familiar voice called out.

Murat looked up and saw Asim, his distant cousin, who was a Partizan commander and a war hero.

'It's me,' Murat said.

'What are you doing here?' Asim demanded.

Murat shrugged.

'I'll get this straightened out,'Asim said and disappeared upstairs.

Five hours later, when Murat had given up hope, Asim returned and escorted him out of the basement. 'Go home.'

Murat began walking, but looked over his shoulder at the basement window, which was visible from the street. The eyes of the other so-called collaborators peered at him.

'What's going to happen to them?' Murat asked.

'Don't ask, Comrade,' Asim told him.

Murat returned home. Later there were rumours that all the other people in the basement had been led to Kozara Mountain, where they had their arms tied behind their backs with wire and were beaten to death by Partizans.

While Murat had been saved from death, he was made to pay. The Communists allocated him a job as a general dogsbody at a hotel, where he spent most of his working life in the basement lugging supplies back and forth to the first floor. Murat never got to achieve his dream of building a large house for his family on the plot of land his father had bequeathed him. Instead he raised his family of five children in a two-bedroom house, and he became worn down by a lifetime of grinding poverty and manual labour. This was the fate that Izet had escaped by marrying Mum.

When Mum was released from hospital she and Izet repaired their fragile relationship, but Izet never felt at ease in the house that my father had bought and paid with his life insurance. It became another indignity that this 'shit' country had foisted upon him. He decided that he wanted to sell it and buy another house – a house that would be his just as much as hers.

He slowly continued the house renovations, gutting the bathroom and installing all new fixtures, replastering and retiling the walls. It took him six months to complete the renovations and in that time we had to use the outside toilet and shower in the bungalow using a portable camp shower.

'When I finish the renovations we'll be able to sell the house,' he said. 'Then we can buy a new house together.'

Mum nodded, feeling conflicted. While she knew he wanted them to make a new start together, this house was all she had ever known and she was nervous about another change.

Izet scoured the local newspapers, circling the houses that he liked and wanted to buy. 'We'd have to get one on a main road. That would be safer from robbers.'

Mum nodded, even though she didn't want to hear the throbbing sound of cars day and night.

When Izet finished the renovations they contacted a real estate agent to value the property. 'Is that all?' Izet demanded when the agent gave them a figure.

'It's a recession at the moment and the market is flat,' the agent said.

'What if we wait for the market to recover?' Mum asked.

'Then you would have to pay more for another house, and with stamp duty and other costs, you'd probably have to take out a loan to cover the difference.'

The only way they would be able to buy a new house was if Izet got a full time job. When we first arrived he attempted working, but as Mum's manic episodes increased he needed to stay home to care for her.

Mum went to see Dr Keddy, seeking some support so that she wouldn't have another breakdown, and returned with a solution. 'Dr Keddy said that you can apply for a carer's pension,' she told Izet.

'What does that mean?' he asked.

'It means that you would get a pension for caring for me – money that would be yours.'

Dr Keddy helped them fill out the forms and they submitted the paperwork. After a few months they were approved and he received his first pension.

Mum thought she had found a solution to their marital problems. Now that they were financially secure and Izet had his own pension, he couldn't complain – and yet he did. In Bosnia, Izet had dreamt of another life elsewhere, feeling constantly dissatisfied. Now that he was elsewhere, he wanted to be anywhere but here.

Their relationship was characterised by her sufferance and his grumbling, culminating in her breakdown and hospitalisation, the cycle unbroken.

CRAZY WOMAN

While the domestic war raged inside the walls of our St Albans home, war was splintering Yugoslavia into six independent states.

For years after we returned to Australia I dreamt of Bosnia. In my dreams I floated above my grandparents' house and settled onto the balcony on the roof where we sat in summer while my grandparents drank coffee, a blanket strewn over the hot concrete. I took off again, floating over the backyard and the verdant garden where I had spent hours planting, weeding and harvesting vegetables, and over the canal that I had skated on in winter in my rubber boots, and soon I was going higher and higher until all I could see below me was the patchwork of green that was my mother's hometown of Bosanska Gradiška.

There was talk of war in Bosnia long before it actually arrived in 1992, but I ignored the hushed conversations between my parents and their visitors, assuming it was hyperbole. When the first news reports broke that the war had begun we collected around the television and watched in disbelief the images of civilians holding rifles, people lying dead on cosmopolitan streets where once they'd drunk coffee and shopped.

The country that was known as Yugoslavia had been a hotbed of tension since the death of President Tito in 1980. Tito, a benevolent dictator, was the glue that held together the six socialist republics that formed the country. I visited his grave for a school excursion, standing before the marble tomb in the museum. I didn't quite understand why this man was so revered, his photo on display in every living room, and why we had come to stare at what was effectively a marble box.

He was the leader of the Partizans, who waged a guerilla liberation war against the Axis and their collaborators, the Serbian royalist Chetniks and the Croatian nationalist Ustaše, during World War II. After the war he created Yugoslavia, and it was his socialist principles – which focused on nationalist interests over religious and ethnic loyalties – that kept the country prosperous and peaceful.

After Tito's death the tensions bubbled to the surface. Each republic wanted its independence, and some of them wanted to claim territories to expand their borders. The international community recognised the secession and independence of the republics in 1992, but Serbia declared war on Bosnia, embarking on a campaign of ethnic cleansing against the Bosniaks (Bosnian Muslims) by establishing concentration camps to starve Bosnian men, rape camps where they committed genocidal rape to impregnate Bosniak women, and mass genocide against Bosniak populations like the one in Srebrenica, where they killed 8,000 Bosniak men and boys.

My mother's hometown, Bosanska Gradiška, was vulnerable due to its position on the right bank of the Sava River, which marked the border between Bosnia and Croatia. My grandparents and extended family clung to their houses as Serbians displaced from Croatia descended. Serbian troops forced Bosniaks to give up their homes to house these Serbian refugees. Soon the Bosniaks were in danger of extermination

– Serbs coveted their houses and land and were not averse to bombings, beatings and extortion to acquire them.

As we watched the media reports of Serb atrocities and waited for news about our family, I felt disconnected from it all. I felt guilty that I was living well while my extended family was suffering, but most of the time I was able to push away thoughts of war and concentrate on the business of living.

It was Mum who felt the strain. She would be washing dishes and suddenly an image of a father being forced to rape his daughter would leap into her mind. She would be folding the washing and then be transported to a concentration camp, surrounded by emaciated men and adolescent boys slowly dying.

My stepfather dealt with his fear differently. He would shout at the television, cursing the Serbs for their vile acts, cursing the Americans for their impotence, cursing the international community for standing by.

'They said it would never happen again,' Izet shouted at the television. 'They said that after the Jews were slaughtered they would never stand by and watch and look at them now.' He spat on the living room floor, expletives filling the air.

Intellectually Mum knew that my stepfather would never raise his hand against her, but hearing the rage in his voice, seeing his whole body contorted with anger, she would become paralysed with fear. Afterwards she was sore and aching: the hours of being clenched fatigued her muscles, making her feel as if she had run a marathon.

At night Mum struggled to sleep and lay in bed, her whole body twitching, until desperate for relief she would get up and clean the house, the television on in the background, waiting for a news bulletin and any mention of the Balkans.

A few days later we were watching television.

'Shut up, asshole,' Izet swore as Bill Clinton spoke at a press conference.

'It's all right, I'll deal with him.' Mum stood and began dancing around the room, waving her skirt around as she listened to music only she could hear. 'This is how I will seduce Clinton.'

Izet was sitting on the couch now, watching her with a perplexed expression. 'Sit down, *Stara*. Sit and calm yourself.'

Mum sat next to him, but soon the urge to move overcame her again. 'I know, I will recite my poetry: "We stand alone, we have no country of our own, briefly we were known, but soon we will be gone." My words will bring world peace, there will be peace for the whole world.' As Mum kept talking her voice rose in volume and soon she was shouting, spittle flying from her mouth as the poetry came to her, unfurling in her mind like a beautiful ribbon. She could see it all, the way her words would travel from her mouth and into the ears of Clinton and all the world leaders. They would be bowed under the weight of her stanzas, their hearts breaking from the beauty of her poetry, tears flowing from their eyes as they felt the pain of Bosnians, and they would act.

'I will save us all,' she shouted, seeing the ribbon stretching from person to person, from Serb to Croat to Bosnian, joining them all together, until religion was washed away and they were once again all brothers and sisters of Adam and Eve, all equal, all children of one God, all full of love in their hearts, and it would all begin with her poem. When she told Izet she expected him to be as happy as she was. There would be no more death, no more pain, no more fear, but instead she found him looking at her with sadness.

'Fatima, you're getting sick,' he said gently.

'No, you're wrong.' Mum shook her head. 'I have finally found my purpose. I have special powers – you just have to believe in my words and everything I tell you will come true.'

'How are you going to reach Clinton?'

'I don't need to – my words will float and find him.' For a moment as she spoke she felt like she was having an out-of-body experience: she could see herself from above, see the bright, shiny eyes, the manic movements, the way her tongue felt thick when she spoke, and then in the next moment she was back in her body, but now her certainty was shaken.

'I think we need to call Vera.'

'No, don't call her,' Mum said, but she sounded doubtful.

'I'll call her to come and talk to you.' Izet gently squeezed her hand.

Mum nodded. As he spoke on the phone she began dancing again. Soon Vera came with a few other professionals. Mum resisted their advice, but seeing my stepfather's sadness and defeat, she finally agreed to be admitted as an informal patient.

Because of the war our whole extended family was transplanted to Australia and resettled as refugees, all of them renting units and flats in St Albans, within walking distance of each other. Twenty-three years after my mother left her homeland, her homeland came to her.

St Albans had always had a large migrant population from the Balkans and this swelled further after the war. Walking to school through the centre of St Albans I would hear my native tongue spoken on the streets. New shops catering to the expanding population sprung up and a sense of community developed between the first wave of migrants and the refugees, but this alliance was uneasy. There were four million Bosnians living in Bosnia, while the Bosnian diaspora was close to two million, with nearly 10,000 settling in Victoria. As the Bosnians came to Australia, so did their old-fashioned attitudes towards mental illness.

On a visit to my grandparents, Mum arrived to find that her sister Nermina was there, as well as a couple from her old neighbourhood. The woman seemed to be glancing at her strangely, and she flinched each time Mum reached for her *fildžan* or leaned in her direction. Mum began to feel self-conscious, but tried to convince herself that she was imagining it. Mum went to the kitchen to take back the coffee tray and upon her return she heard the woman ask my Tetka Nermina, 'Are you sure I have nothing to be scared of?' Mum realised that her suspicions were correct: the woman was afraid of her.

Mum returned to the living room and her sister beckoned her over.

'I'm sorry I'm being strange today,' the woman told Mum. 'My auntie has schizophrenia. One day she was having an episode and she cornered me and tried to kill me, so I'm scared you'll hurt me.'

'Of course she won't hurt you.' Tetka Nermina put an arm around Mum's shoulders.

Mum shook her head and tried to force a smile, but her face felt frozen. They all sat back down, but Mum couldn't sit still. Her chest felt tight and her skin prickled. 'I'm not feeling well,' she finally murmured and left. As she walked home she took deep breaths, trying to ease the tightness in her chest.

It became hard for her to visit people, even her family.

Every time she was out among other Bosnians she kept feeling their glances and questioned what they were thinking when they looked at her. Did they fear her? Did they worry that she would snap and hurt them? Once this thought was planted in her mind it seemed to mushroom and take all the oxygen from her. It became hard to breathe when she was outside. Soon she stopped leaving her house. It was ironic that Mum had spent her whole life as an exile from her homeland, and then when her homeland came to her she was exiled again.

'I'm scared that I will hurt someone,' she told Vera.

'Why do you think that?' Vera asked, exchanging a concerned look with my stepfather.

'I'm just scared,' Mum said. She began crying and Vera held out a box of tissues.

'This stupid woman put the thought in her head,' Izet said, explaining what had happened. 'I keep telling her not to think about it, but she just can't let it go.'

Mum clutched the tissue in her hand. 'I don't think I will hurt anyone, but sometimes when I'm visiting my parents and there's a new person there, the thought pops into my head.' It seemed like the more she tried to not think about it, the more it happened, and each time it did she struggled to breathe.

'I think you're getting panic attacks,' Vera said, after Mum described her symptoms. 'Do you feel like this at any other time?'

'When Izet leaves the house, I get anxious,' Mum admitted.

For years Izet had only left the house for errands: to buy groceries, to pay bills, or to attend to car repairs or registrations. He kept buying, repairing and replacing the car, each time looking for something better. The only social outings he had were visits to friends and family with Mum, but then he started dressing nicely and going to the coffee shop. For a while Mum had thought that perhaps he was having an affair, until my Tetka confirmed that he was at the local Bosnian coffee shop with her brother-in-law Damir and other Bosnians. Soon he got sick of their humour and began frequenting coffee shops where he wouldn't see any Bosnians.

'Do you know why you feel like this?' Vera probed.

'I worry that he won't come back.'

My stepfather kept reassuring her that he just wanted some alone time, but she knew the truth. He wanted to be alone without her. Each time he left the house she felt her breath catch, and while he was gone she wondered whether he would return.

'Why do you worry that he won't come back?'

'I treated him badly when I was sick. Tried to kick him out. Now he thinks that I don't want to be with him.'

Mum had broken the unspoken covenant of their relationship. Izet never said he wanted to leave her; instead, he always talked about wanting to leave this shit country. She had wondered where his rage came from until Vera suggested that he was projecting all his anger and frustration onto Australia.

The fact that she had tried to kick him out, even though she had been under the influence of her illness, proved the unevenness of their relationship. She was the one who had the upper hand. It was her house, her pension, her country, and he was just a visitor in her world. All she had to do was rescind the invitation and he was left with nothing.

'Do you want to leave?' Vera asked Izet.

'I'm not leaving. We're married,' Izet said.

Mum nodded, trying to believe him.

'We need to work on your breathing to calm you down. I'll give you some meditation tapes.' As Vera prepared a care plan to deal with her anxiety Mum nodded along, taking deep breaths.

I was facing my own battles because of the war in Bosnia. I had grown up with parents who followed the few markers of Muslim faith that Bosnians followed: circumcising male children and giving their children Muslim names. Some Bosnians drank alcohol, some didn't. Some ate pork, others didn't. While my father drank alcohol, we never ate pork in our family. Many Bosnians were members of the Communist Party, including my grandfather. Not many people prayed and only older women covered their hair. Growing up I knew that I was Bosnian, but had called myself Yugoslav. I thought of my religion as secondary; instead, it was my first language and geographical location that marked my identity in Australia.

As a child, being Muslim meant dressing up in our finest clothes and spending the day at mosque with other Bosnians. Using the magical phrase '*Bajram Barićula*' and offering my hand, I received cash from family friends. Come Christmas time, though, when all my schoolfriends talked about what they'd received from Santa, I ran home asking where my Christmas presents were. 'We don't celebrate Christmas,' Mum explained. 'We're Muslims and you receive money during *Bajram* instead.'

She tried to convince me money was much better, but those golden days of collecting money and buying sweets from the milk bar until my stomach ached were long gone from my memory. All I knew was that I was different and I vibrated with desire for the toys that my friends bragged about, the Cabbage Patch doll I dreamt about and never owned.

When I lived with my grandparents in Yugoslavia I was sent to religious school, *Mejtef*, to learn about Islam. Ideological restrictions had relaxed in the five years since President Tito had died. While I eventually forgot most of the lectures from the *Hodža*, one perfect moment was indelibly imprinted in my mind and shaped my spirituality. 'Allah is all-seeing and all-knowing. He has no shape, and no form. He is in the sky, in the earth, and in us,' the *Hodža* lectured as he walked up and down the class.

I was overcome by this. In Australia, a Christian country, God was portrayed with statues and paintings of Jesus Christ as a man, but now this new image took over and something clicked into place. God became a secret companion who was always with me, guiding me. 'There is the world we see and the world we don't see,' the *Hodža* continued. And as I got older I had the opportunity to confirm this notion that there were things in this world we didn't see and couldn't touch that existed just beyond our realm.

Now that Yugoslavia had broken apart, I wasn't Yugoslav anymore – now I was Bosnian. Because of the atrocities perpetrated by Serbs, the Western world now knew that Bosnians were Muslims. When questions of ethnicity entered the conversation and I said I was Yugoslav, strangers would demand more information. Was I Bosnian, Croatian or Serbian? When I told them I was Bosnian more questions followed: Why was the war happening? Why didn't I cover my hair? And most importantly, how was it that there were Muslims smack dab in the middle of Europe?

While I was struggling with this perception of myself outside my home and community, I was also battling the expectations being placed on me by Mum and our extended family. Mum wanted me to attend *Mejtef*, and there was even talk of me and Haris going to a newly established Muslim school in Werribee, but I soon nixed that.

With the Bosnian diaspora invading St Albans there were other effects. We were under scrutiny in a way that we hadn't been before.

One day I came home from school and Mum greeted me with the question, 'Who was the boy you were kissing?'

'What are you talking about?' I demanded. I had firmly avoided all romantic entanglements at my new high school and hadn't exchanged saliva with a boy in over a year.

She named a newly arrived migrant who had called Mum a few minutes before. Apparently she had seen me in front of Woolworths in St Albans, kissing a boy.

I was stunned for a moment until I remembered that I'd bumped into a male friend of the family and we had kissed on the cheek when we parted, a custom that all Bosnians followed when greeting or taking leave of acquaintances and family. When I explained this to Mum she just nodded, but I was outraged.

I was once again under surveillance by the Bosnian spy network, and any and all infractions would be reported and gossiped about. I was expected to have Bosnian friends and to marry a Bosnian, so I promptly vowed to break both these expectations.

CONFESSION

Because my father died overseas and we never saw his body, there was always a feeling of incompleteness surrounding his death. Even though we'd been at his grave I imagined that there had been a mistake and the wrong man had been buried in his place. I never thought he was really gone; instead, he was on holiday and one day he would return.

Growing up, my favourite TV show was *The Six Million Dollar Man* starring Lee Majors. In the show Majors's character is rebuilt with bionic limbs and implants and he becomes an intelligence agent. In every episode he performs heroic deeds, saving someone with his new superpowers.

One of my fantasies was that my father had experienced the same fate and he wasn't really dead, but had instead been remade into a half-man, half-robot and one day there would be a knock on the door and there he would be.

Mum had this exact same feeling. One day she started laughing to herself, and I turned around and asked why.

'Nothing – I'm just remembering a story your dad told me.' She laughed again.

I stared at her and waited. I was always curious to learn about my father. From as far back as I could remember she had drip-fed me stories about him. He was the firstborn and had been terribly spoiled by his mother. He had a younger brother who was overlooked and tormented by him. One time when his younger brother transgressed in some way he punished him by holding his hands on the stovetop until blisters formed.

While I knew chances were this story would be no better than the ones that had preceded it, I was still always curious to know about my father. He was a mystery that I would never solve. In my adolescence I'd tried to find out about who he really was, collecting stories from my father's friends, but he was never a real person to me, just an amalgamation of strange tales and contradictory anecdotes.

What I did know for a fact was that my father came from a small village in the Bosnian highlands surrounded by an emerald green forest populated by bears and wolves. When trouble found you there was no one for miles.

His village was perched on top of a hill, it and required a strong constitution to trek up and down the well-worn paths linking it to the *granap* at the bottom. Next to the *granap* was a bus stop that went to the nearest city of Travnik, an hour away.

Mum wavered for a moment. 'There was a mute girl in your father's village,' she finally said. 'Your father told me a funny story about her.'

The movie I'd been watching was quickly forgotten and I'd turned towards her, curious to know where this tale was leading. I remembered the mute girl from my one and only visit to my father's village and Mum crying as she forced a hug upon the girl and whispered something in her ear.

My father was the handsome Casanova of the hamlet, and it wasn't long before the mute girl succumbed to his charms. My father bragged to his friend Davud about his latest conquest, and this planted the seed of an idea in Davud's head.

As Mum recounted the story to me I wondered how it had all gone down. Was the mute girl walking along when Davud saw her? Did he try to engage her in conversation, asking her where she was going, perhaps offering a compliment? Or perhaps he saw her walking alone and stepped in behind her. Something in the stealthy way he followed her would have set off her internal alarm. She wanted to speed up and get away from him, but an internal instinct warned that to do so would only provoke the predator within.

She counted her footsteps, fighting to overcome her panic. She only had a few hundred metres until the forest ended and then they would be in a wide-open meadow where the sun lit up the golden fields. On the other side of the field were houses and safety. Suddenly she was yanked by the arm. As she struggled, her vocal cords were able to produce only grunts, rough hands pinched her flesh in their grasp. Her world tilted as she was lifted off the ground; her eyes looked up at the canopy of trees above her, the wind making them dance.

She was thrown on the ground, her arms held down, while her legs were yanked open and her flesh was prodded. Piercing pain cut through her and all she could do was close her eyes until it was over.

I was back in the darkened living room, sitting in the middle of the floor. I felt vertigo as I tried to process the story my mother had told me.

'Davud raped the mute girl. Your father laughed when he told me.' Mum laughed to herself. 'He said, "It wasn't like she could tell anyone."'

An ill feeling overcame me and I fought nausea. 'It's not funny,' I shouted at the stranger who was my mother. I had been on the receiving end of men's lecherous attentions and found them nothing to laugh about.

When I was thirteen years old I travelled by bus to the shopping centre in Keilor Downs, which had the only bookstore within travelling distance of my house. I had taken this bus regularly since I had discovered my favourite romance novelist a year earlier. I was collecting her backlist and each time I saved up $12.95 I would make the trek. Usually I would run from the bookshop and begin reading as soon I as I reached the bus stop. I would only stop reading long enough to get off bus and walk home, but the wait to get back to the world of cynical heroes and dainty heroines was agony.

The bus was crowded and a man sat down next to me. I was staring out the window, fixated on the thought of buying my next novel and how desperately I wanted to read it.

It was a warm summer day and the man was wearing shorts. His hairy sweaty knee pressed up against mine and I shifted away. I glanced at him and saw that he was staring straight ahead. The aisle was full of people holding onto the seat handles behind us, slightly leaning in, pushing him towards me.

I began to feel uncomfortable. I didn't like men sitting next to me, especially not so close, but we were turning into the road where the shopping centre was. I only had three more stops to endure and then I could get off and get my book.

I turned back to the window when I felt his leg again. I glanced at the man. He was still staring straight ahead, his face blank and uninterested. I frowned. Then I felt it properly. There was no mistaking what it was. It was a hand. A hand was on my knee. I glanced at the guy – he was still staring straight ahead, blank-faced.

I didn't want to believe it. I was imagining it. It was a hot day. There wasn't really a hand on my knee. The hand moved up. I began hyperventilating. I didn't know what to do. Should I shout? Should I scream? There were all these people around, but I was alone and very scared. Why was this happening to me?

He took my lack of movement as approval. The hand moved again, and I snapped out of my inertia. It was just about to touch my vagina. I stood up and pulled the cord, running off the bus like I was being chased.

As I watched it drive away, my fear retreated as anger took its place. Now I would have to walk for an extra fifteen minutes to get to the shopping centre. I was angry with the man who had molested me, but I was more angry with myself for sitting there and taking it. Why hadn't I spoken up? The bus was full of people. All I had to do was shout and scream so everyone would know what he was doing, but I'd been too scared about the embarrassment I would cause. I didn't want to face the truth of what was going on, and rather than accepting it, I tried to talk myself out of it. I promised myself I would never make that mistake again.

When I was fifteen years old I was walking home from Veronica's house at night by myself. She lived a kilometre away. We didn't go to the same high school, so we visited each other nearly every day after school and had sleepovers most weekends. It was the summer school holidays and I would stay later and later, sometimes until nine o'clock.

Veronica's mother drove me home a few times, not feeling comfortable about letting me walk home so late, but she worked night shift as a nurse and was getting tired of driving me.

I called my parents and asked my stepfather to pick me up. Mum wasn't happy with him being my chauffeur and said that he couldn't come so I'd got into the habit of making my own way home.

I was walking down Veronica's street towards Main Road when a boy rode past on a bike. He passed me and went up the street, before doing U-turn and returning to ride beside me. Unease filled me.

'Psssst,' he called.

I looked over. He was riding slowly, one hand holding the handlebars steady, the other on his penis as he masturbated.

I sped up, but he kept shadowing me.

Fear gripped me. The street was dark and deserted; we were the only two people around. The streetlights barely penetrated the gloom. I was on the left-hand side of the street, walking alongside my former high school, which stretched for most of the block. On the other side of the street, all the houses were closed off by thick dark curtains. No one would hear me if I screamed.

I reached the gym building and the car park, and was a few steps away from the great stretch of oval. I could hear the boy's thoughts as if they were floating in the darkness with us. There was no one around, and there was nowhere for me to run. All he had to do was jump off the bike and throw me over the waist-high mesh fence, an easy feat with my slight build. Then we would be on the grassy oval, hidden from view from anyone who passed by.

I only had a minute or two until he made his move. I looked around for options. If I ran it would incite him more. He was on a bike and could chase me down. I could run to someone's house, but they were all on the other side of the street, and I would have to pass him. Time was running out. Another step or two and I would be completely open to danger.

A light came on down the street. There were voices. A family were seeing out their guests. The boy stopped.

I shouted at the top of my lungs, 'Get the fuck away from me, you pervert.' I kept shouting even as he rode off.

As soon as he was far enough away, I ran. I ran every single step home, bursting through the front door out of breath and in a panic.

'A boy attacked me,' I gasped. 'He was on his bike and he flashed himself at me.'

My mother's face closed down with guilt.

'I'll fix him,' my brother said and left the house.

He collected a posse of his mates and they drove around looking. They found a boy who was riding a bike near a milk bar close to Veronica's house, but they weren't sure if he was the one. How could they be? I didn't see his face. He was only a menacing shadow on a bicycle.

I had learnt to assess and react to danger, and I had saved myself with the power of my voice, but the mute girl had had none.

'It's not fucking funny at all,' I shouted at Mum again, my eyes burning with tears.

'Of course not.' Mum sat up straight, the smile fading from her face. 'When I saw the mute girl I told her I was sorry for what happened to her.'

'Then why were you laughing?' I demanded.

'It's the way he told it,' she said. 'He made it sound like a joke.'

'But it's not a joke.' I ran to my bedroom and locked the door. I spent the afternoon hugging my pillow as I cried.

She spent the afternoon apologising, trying to make me understand that her laughter was not because she found the story funny, but it was too late.

Her laughter was probably a nervous reaction – she was in the grip of mania, and her illness lowered her inhibitions – but I became stuck in that moment when I learnt that my father thought a woman's rape was a joke. That was the night I stopped my nightly prayers, and for months afterwards I struggled to fall asleep without this ritual. It was also the night that I turned away from Mum and the stories that had once kept me enthralled.

Years later I told Mum how her stories of my father had made me feel and guilt coloured her face. She began telling me other stories. 'He loved you so much,' she'd say. 'It was never too hard for him to change your nappy or give you your bottle, and you know what Bosnian men are like.'

And when she said that I remembered the one photo of my childhood I cherished. In it I am one year old and have just started to walk. My father is chasing after me, his hands outstretched as he tries to catch me before I fall, the expression on his face one I see on my husband's face as he looks at our daughter. It is a look of pride and adoration.

RUNAWAY

'Hey, put that back, *mala*,' my stepdad said, as I snatched the remote and changed the channel. *Mala* was his nickname for me – 'little girl'.

'No,' I said. '*Booker* is about to start.'

At fifteen I was boy crazy and had spent the afternoon in feverish anticipation of my favourite TV show. It was a spin-off from *21 Jump Street*, an incredibly unrealistic cop show that featured gorgeous young police officers going undercover in high schools. *Booker* had Richard Grieco, the object of my latest crush. I had his posters on my wall with lipstick marks all over them and had even sent a letter to his fan club, receiving a signed photo for my efforts.

'I was watching that doco,' Izet said.

I ignored him, keeping my back to him. We had only one television and it was a source of constant battles between Izet, Haris and me; Mum hardly got a look in.

Izet took back the remote control and switched the channel.

'Put it back,' I yelled. 'It's about to start!'

'Amra,' Mum said. 'It's Izet's turn to watch.'

'But it's *Booker* …'

'You can't always get to watch what you want,' Mum said calmly. 'You have to share. You watched *Quantum Leap* yesterday and Izet didn't watch his show.'

'You always take his side!' I shouted. 'You know I love this TV show and I watch it every week. He shouldn't be watching this crap anyway.' I pointed at the documentary on the screen.

Usually at this point my stepdad would crumble and tell Mum to let it go, but it was true – I had been hogging the TV. I had a roster of television shows I was completely incapable of giving up.

'I told you, it's his turn.' Mum changed the channel.

I got up and switched the channel again using the buttons below the screen. The theme song – 'Hot in the City', sung by Billy Idol – was playing and I felt the familiar wave of excitement at seeing my crush on screen. I swayed to the beat and rubbed my hands together.

The channel changed again. 'What the fuck did you do that for?' I yelled. My stepdad was sitting on the couch with the remote in his hand. 'I fucking told you I was watching that!' I continued ranting, uttering all sorts of profanity, while Izet adopted a turtle pose, his only defence to my adolescent rage.

'Amra, enough,' Mum said. 'Go to your room.'

'No!' I stood in front of the television so Izet couldn't watch. This, for me, was more than a battle over the television – I was really fighting for Mum's attention. It seemed that she always sided with Izet, proving that she loved him more. The rejection fuelled my rage.

'Go to your room or I'm going to get the *oklagija*,' Mum said. This was a long rolling pin that resembled a broom handle, which was used to make pita.

I switched the channel and sat back down in front of the TV. Usually Mum didn't hit me – the threat alone would be enough for me to listen – but on this night my lust for Richard Grieco overpowered my fear.

Mum hit me lightly on the head from behind with the *oklagija*. It was more like a tap, but that didn't matter to me.

'You fucking hit me!' I shouted, crying. 'How dare you hit me?' I ran to my bedroom, slamming the door and crying furiously, messily. I felt rejected. The pain of it ripped through me. She didn't love me. She had never loved me and this proved it.

Mum knocked on the door: 'Come back. We've changed the channel. You can watch your show.'

I wavered for a moment. Of course I wanted to perve on Richard Grieco, but I wasn't going to give her the satisfaction. She'd hit me. She was going to pay for this.

'No, I don't want anything to do with you!' I shouted. 'I fucking hate you both.'

I heard Mum's footsteps retreat from the door. I opened my window and jumped out. I wheeled my bicycle from the backyard and rode the five kilometres to Zehra's house. She had moved out of the share house and was living by herself in a bungalow behind a house in Sunshine.

There were no lights on, and when I knocked she didn't answer the door. I didn't want to go home so I settled on her front step to wait. An hour passed and I was flagging. Then I heard a car pull up outside the house. Zehra appeared through the side gate, accompanied by a man. They stopped to kiss and I shuffled my feet in embarrassment, not sure whether I should interrupt or not.

The man saw me and pushed Zehra away. She looked at me over her shoulder. 'What are you doing here?'

'I ran away from home. Mum hit me on the head.' I was crying again.

She hesitated. 'I guess you'd better come in then.' She unlocked the door. 'This is Milan.'

Her bungalow was tiny. When you walked in there was a kitchen and a shower, then you climbed a few steps into a space that was at most five metres by two metres. There was a television, a couch and a cane chair, and behind a cane screen was her bed. She'd painted all her cane furniture glossy black and accessorised with dashes of pink.

'We've got to call Mum.' Zehra took me to the phone box around the corner.

I didn't want to call her – I wanted her, and my stepfather, to suffer – but then Zehra would get in trouble. Mum agreed to let me stay the night and said they would come by tomorrow to pick me up.

Back at Zehra's I sat across from Milan, checking him out while Zehra made coffee. 'So what happened?' Zehra sat down at the table after passing Milan his mug.

'I hate her and I hate living there.' I picked at the laminate on the side of the table. 'I can't wait to get out of there.'

'But you've still got another three years at least, so you'd better find a way to make the best of it.' Zehra squeezed my hand.

I sighed. I felt like I was a prisoner and freedom was too far away to reach.

The next morning Mum came by. Her lips tightened in displeasure and anger, and she kept her eyes away from me as if I didn't exist. She and Zehra and my stepdad spoke in the bungalow while I waited outside. When they finished, Izet and Mum left without saying a word to me.

'What happened?' I asked, deflated. Of all the reactions I'd expected, this wasn't it.

'Mum agreed to let you stay here for the weekend. Give everyone a chance to cool down,' Zehra said as we went back inside.

It was as I had suspected. They didn't want me around. Over the next few months my rage intensified and I sought to escape my parents with weekend sleepovers with Zehra and my best friend Veronica.

I can't remember Veronica before the fateful day in Year Seven when we became friends. I know we used to hang out in a group together, but she was always shy and didn't speak much, so she blended into the background. Our friendship formed because of my boy craziness.

I had developed a crush on Dragon, whose real name was Dragan, a Year Ten boy who was very much desired by all the girls because of his pretty face and glossy brown hair that touched his collarbone. I had discovered his address and phone number through the phone book and used to stalk him, hiding out on the street and walking past his house, desperately seeking a glimpse of him. I would crank-call him throughout the day just to hear his voice, and was sometimes brave enough to say a few words and start a conversation, before quickly hanging up in embarrassment.

At school I followed him around the grounds, and committed acts of ever increasing desperation to attract his attention. Some of my tokens of affection met with more success than others. When I presented him with a badge I'd bought that said *Smile if you're sexy*, he pinned it to his chest and smiled every time I passed. He wasn't impressed when I threw his backpack on the roof of the walkway and threatened to dob me in to the teacher if I didn't retrieve it.

Our biology teacher had organised a dissection. The class was put into pairs and the teacher gave each pair a frozen rat preserved in a plastic bag of formaldehyde. Squeals of disgust and gagging sounds filled the classroom as the teacher instructed us how to open the sealed bag and proceed with dissecting the rat. Some of the tough boys abandoned their dissections and hid out in the corridor, but I calmly followed the teacher's instructions. Four years of living in Bosnia had given me a cast-iron stomach. I enjoyed the fact that my more squeamish classmates were looking at me askance.

'All right, thank you everyone for your maturity and cooperation,' the teacher said as we completed our lesson. 'I'm going to come around and collect the rats. Please don't think about keeping a memento for yourselves.' She carefully checked each rat as she collected it, ensuring that all its body parts were present.

I looked at my rat lying on the table, specifically at its long tail, and a terrible thought formed. When the teacher came by I held the body of the rat and the tail in one hand so it looked like the tail was still attached. As I dropped the rat into the bucket, I tucked the severed tail into my sleeve, using the sleight of hand from my shoplifting days in Bosnia. As the teacher continued around the room, I put the tail in my pocket, looking forward to the props I'd get in the schoolyard for my daring.

At lunchtime I went to the oval with my posse. Dragon and his friends slowly nudged their way towards us. This was the first time he had voluntarily come towards me; usually he was my sun and I the planet that orbited around his hemisphere. I put my hand in my pocket and the devil took hold of me.

'I have a rat's tail,' I said. As I had expected, all eyes turned to me. I noticed disbelief on Dragon's face. I retrieved the tail, swinging it in the air in front of me.

'It's not real,' one of the boys shouted. I stopped swinging it and held it still so they could see it. They came closer, examining the rings and the way it thinned to a point in my hands.

'Fuck, it's a rat's tail,' Dragon's friend, Tom, said. He looked at me with new-found respect.

Emboldened, I flicked the tail. The girls shrieked and ran away; the boys flinched, quickly correcting themselves and not moving further. I ran at Dragon with the tail. He started to run away before turning back and wrapping his arms around me, holding my arm away from him. He lifted me onto the fence and started lowering me to the ground. 'Promise you won't try to touch me with the tail, or I'll drop you.'

I was laughing, the feel of his hands on me filling me with joy. Everyone had come back and they were laughing as they watched us.

The girls shrieked, 'Drop her, drop her.'

'I promise,' I blurted out through spurts of laughter.

He lifted me and put me on the ground. I was about to learn there would be a high price to pay for capturing his attention.

The next day I was doing my usual Dragon stalking when his friend approached me.

'Dragon wants to get on with you,' Tom told me.

I froze. This was the total opposite of what I wanted – I had picked Dragon for his unattainability. He only went with the cool girls and I was anything but.

'Why would he want to kiss Rat Girl?' I heard one his mates ask snidely, and I wondered the same thing myself.

I followed Tom to the PE building, where Dragon was standing by the emergency exit door. He had jammed some paper into the doorframe during his PE class and now he opened it and took my hand. I followed him inside. We were at the bottom of a stairway. When he closed the door it was pitch black.

We found each other by touch. Dragon was much taller and his hands rested on my shoulders. We began kissing, but the height difference was too big. He sat down and pulled me onto his lap. As we kissed his hands were all over my body. Squeezing, probing, stroking. I stiffened, hating the way he touched me, but I felt I had no right to complain. I had brought this on myself by stalking him. I had given him the signal he could do what he wanted.

I don't know how long we were there for, but it was a long time and to me it felt like an eternity. Each touch was torturous. He took my silence for compliance and became bolder, his hand moving to my crotch. He tugged on the zip. I flinched, pushing his hands away. He changed direction, squeezing my buttocks.

He stopped and I felt his breath on my neck as he panted. 'We should get back.'

I nodded, but realised it was too dark for him to see. 'Okay,' I whispered. I stood and adjusted my clothes, hearing a rustle as he did the same.

When we walked out the light was blinding and I felt dazed to be free. My friends demanded salacious details, but I stood mute with horror. Somehow Veronica came to my side and she walked me off school grounds. I told her what had happened, words jerking out of me in a shameful whisper. I started crying and the feelings of shame and humiliation built in my throat, choking me.

'What do you want to do?' Veronica asked.

'Run.'

'Let's run.'

We ran the length of the block and with each step I felt a release. And just like that my crush died a swift and sudden death, and my friendship with Veronica was born.

I loved sleeping over at Veronica's house, and even though her parents called her out to help with household chores, they mostly left us alone in her room. At home, Mum spent most of the day sleeping on the couch in her tracksuit pants, rising only long enough to complete the essential household tasks she was required to do. I didn't know at the time that she was experiencing the other side of bipolar, and that the medication she took to bring her out of the manic phase was flattening her.

Whenever Veronica came over to my house Mum would come knocking on the door and sit between us on my bed.

'I found out about Eldin's family,' she said. I'd developed a crush on Eldin, a Bosnian boy. Mum had been rapt, saying she would get some intel about him from the Bosnian network.

'I don't care anymore,' I told Mum.

I had seen Eldin at the train station that day. We'd been having a flirtatious conversation when he saw a girl walking past and described her as an aeroplane, forming his hands into an hourglass shape. 'Okay, I've got to get going,' he said and left, following the girl onto the carriage.

'I'm sure he didn't mean it,' Mum said when I told her about it. 'He just doesn't speak English well.'

'We were speaking in Bosnian,' I snapped.

She tried again. 'Maybe he just wanted to get a seat on the train and that's why he left so quickly.'

'The train was half empty.'

I was disgusted that she was trying to push a Bosnian onto me. 'You just want me to be a good Bosnian girl so you can trot me out to the community, and you don't care if he's a sleazebag.'

'That's not true. I just want the best for you.'

'Well, I'm not going to take advice from someone who lies on the couch like a beached whale all day.'

Mum's face crumpled, and I was momentarily appalled at the way I was treating her. She was a soft target for malicious comments and I was usually her champion. When the hairdresser wouldn't accept Mum's concession card for the advertised discount, I was the one who called to complain. Her new psychiatrist had started their first session by asking her about her fears, and after she'd shared them he told her she was crazy. Mum came home in tears, and I called and complained about his unprofessional conduct.

'I'll leave you girls to talk.' Mum left, slightly hunched like she was absorbing a blow.

'You were horrible to your mother,' Veronica admonished me after Mum closed the door behind her.

'She's horrible to me.'

'That's not true, and anyway, nothing changes the fact that she's your mother and she deserves your respect.'

I sullenly nodded and the next day I offered a half-hearted apology that Mum accepted. I'd achieved my purpose – Mum didn't interrupt our sleepovers again.

DIAGNOSIS

Many of my childhood friendships were brief, and only one is still bountiful and thriving twenty-eight years after we met – that's with my best friend, Veronica. In my last year of high school, I would have another friendship that would transform my life.

Snežana and I were drawn to each other because we were so alike. We were both the products of our childhoods – slightly damaged and older than our years. Snežana had come from Serbia with her mother when she was a child. When her stepfather became abusive, her mother refused to leave him – it was Snežana who left and became a ward of the state, moving into a shared house funded by the Department of Human Services with other young girls who had nowhere else to go.

Our Western suburbs highschool had no uniform and most students showcased their wares in double denim: denim jackets and jeans, or tracksuit pants. Snežana and I didn't care what others thought about our fashion choices. Snežana once wore a jumper and a tie to school, and she ignored the titters about it. No one wore a tie at our school, not even the teachers, and to wear it with a jumper just seemed the height of absurdity that stirred our peers' demand for conformity. I caused a stir with my op-shop creations – tops with the bottom edge cut off and rips along the shoulder seams to expose my skin.

Our main point of difference was that I wasn't as much of a loner as she was. Outside school I had my best friend Veronica, and at school I was part of a group of both boys and girls. Snežana only had the girls she shared a house with.

A few weeks into our friendship Snežana invited me home. All the furniture in the independent living facility was second-hand, cobbled together by the Department of Human Services, which is why I felt so at home there. It was like our house before the influx of Copperart furniture.

She showed me her bedroom and closed the door. 'This is my inspiration wall.' She pointed at the clippings covering the back of the door.

I stepped closer, reading the poems, quotes and novel extracts. 'Wow, this is amazing. I collect quotes too, but I write them in my diary.'

'This is my favourite poem.' She handed me a book. I sat on her bed and read the verses, feeling the poignancy of the words.

'What do you think?' Snežana asked.

'It's so lonely, and haunting, and beautiful.'

Snežana gave me a rare smile. She was my first friend who loved reading as much I did, and it was such a pleasure to be able to share this part of my life.

'Why would you spend time with that weirdo?' my schoolfriend Jennifer demanded when I told her I'd visited Snežana.

'She's not a weirdo,' I said, heat in my voice. When Jennifer looked sceptical I told her Snežana's life story.

'So she lives on her own?'

'Yes – she can't live at home so she's like a ward of the state. It's really sad.'

'Yeah, it is. You should ask her to come and hang out with us,' Jennifer said.

I was proud that my friends were so accepting. I couldn't wait to get Snežana in our circle. My chance came the next day.

'Come and hang out with us,' I asked Snežana, tugging her towards the front of the school where we hung out.

Snežana shook me off. 'No, I'm going to the library.'

'But I want you to meet my friends.'

'They're your friends,' Snežana said, 'not mine.'

I felt like I'd been slapped, but Snežana's forthrightness was one of the things I liked most about her. Where most of my peers would nod along and then bitch behind each other's backs, Snežana had no such filter.

'Why don't you come with me?' Snežana said. 'You'd be better off reading than spending time with those proles.'

Coming from a communist society, Snežana divided the world into proles and capitalists. (Snežana, of course, belonged to neither category – she was an intellectual who rejected material possessions and her only purpose was learning.)

'Okay.' I wanted to prove to her I was on her intellectual level, so I followed her to the library. She'd come to visit me a few weeks ago and I felt she may have found me wanting.

When she'd walked into my bedroom I saw it through her eyes. The posters of pretty boys with lipstick marks on them. The vanity table covered with feminine paraphernalia. The birthday cards blu-tacked to the mirror as proof of my social life. I knew that Snežana was judging me as a conformist. I wanted to go out on the ledge with her and be a true outsider, someone who didn't give a shit about anything or anyone, who wasn't afraid of going to school with hairy legs and armpits, who didn't obsess about appearance or likeability.

'What are those books?' She'd pointed at the stack of Mills and Boons on my bedside table.

'Oh, just some novels.'

Snežana frowned as she picked one up. She examined the cover and read the blurb. 'Ah, *romantični romani*,' she said. 'You're better than this shallow filth. I'll lend you a book.' She returned the novel to the stack without saying anything more.

She expanded my horizon beyond Mills and Boon. Under her tutelage I read *Wuthering Heights* and became obsessed with Catherine and Heathcliff, including the 1939 movie. When I was at a second-hand bookstore doing my romance novel swap I noticed a hardcover book that I wouldn't usually give a second glance. It was *Myra Breckinridge* by Gore Vidal, published in 1968, its pages yellowed and the spine falling apart. I took it home and read it in one night, obsessed with the diary of Myra, a creation of Myron who is undergoing a clinical sex change. Some might call it pornographic, but something about it spoke to me. This character was an outsider, and the novel connected with me on a visceral level. I knew only one other person who would appreciate it.

'This is an amazing book,' Snežana said after she'd read it. 'Thank you for giving it to me, dear Amra. You are a true friend.'

I smiled. Snežana had learnt English in her early teens; she had a faint accent and a formal way of speaking.

After coming back from Bosnia I'd had to relearn how to speak like an Australian. I used to say 'dance' and 'chance' with a long *a*, like BBC broadcasters used under the influence of an English teacher. I was constantly asked where I was from, because people thought my accent was South African. I learnt to pepper my speech with Aussie slang, and called people 'darl' and 'love' in order to blend in. With Snežana I could speak how I wanted, without worrying that she would tease me as my schoolfriends had.

'Am I able to keep it a little longer? I would like to re-read it.'

'You keep it,' I told her. 'I won't re-read it.'

She smiled and hugged me. Next time I saw the book she had lovingly put contact on the cover, a black and white pattern, and was proudly carrying it from class to class.

A week later I was in the toilets when Snežana burst in, slamming the door behind her. 'I need to talk to you,' she demanded.

'Sure.' I finished wiping my hands on a paper towel. 'I'll see you guys later,' I told my friends, and followed Snežana out into the corridor.

'Why are you talking about me?'

'What are you going on about?' I'd never said a bad word about her and I couldn't understand her animosity.

'You're telling people about me. Telling them my personal things.'

'I didn't tell anyone anything personal,' I said. 'I'm your friend.'

'Then how do they know about my home situation?'

'Well, I told them that –' I began, but she cut me off.

'I can't be friends with someone who doesn't respect my privacy.' She handed me back *Myra Breckinridge* and left.

I walked away feeling flat. I didn't know what had just happened. What had I done that was so wrong?

The next day I had an appointment with Miss Meadowcroft, the school counsellor. I had started seeing her a few months before, when Mum was sick and I'd been staying home to supervise her. The hospital was under pressure and after her last episode Mum had been released home after only a short stay. She was under the supervision of the CATT team, but she couldn't be left alone in case she went on shopping sprees or overstayed her welcome while visiting friends, unaware of how intrusive and rude she was being.

Mum didn't have a good grasp of English so I used to write notes to the teacher about my absences and get Mum to sign it. Because of the medication her handwriting was atrocious – her signature was her name printed in letters that didn't join. It didn't take long for Mum to get better, but by then I didn't want to return to school. I'd write absence notes and fake Mum's signature so I could spend the day in the library, reading to escape my life.

Eventually the coordinators twigged and I was called into the principal's office. Sitting beside me was my Year Nine coordinator, Miss McConnell.

'We need to talk to you about your absences,' the principal began, and I gulped. I was always late for first period and had clocked up fifteen absences.

'We were looking at your absence notes.' He pulled out a stack of them. 'If you see here, this signature looks different to this signature.' He held up a note from the beginning of the year and one at the end. I'd gotten sloppy forging Mum's signature, my cursive handwriting bleeding into her printed signature.

'My mum is sick a lot,' I told him. 'The medication makes her hand shake and these are from when she's better and her hand isn't shaking.'

The principal and Miss McConnell exchanged a look. 'What kind of illness does she have?' he asked.

I told him about Mum's nervous breakdowns and that I had to take care of her.

'Thank you, Amra,' he said when I finished. 'We'll call your mother to confirm what you've told us.'

I spent the rest of the day in a state of feverish anticipation and then flew home. 'Has the principal called you?' I demanded as I ran into the living room, out of breath. Mum shook her head. I told her about being called into the principal's office. 'You have to cover for me,' I told her. 'You have to tell them that you signed all the notes.'

Mum's face had tightened as I spoke. I didn't have to explain to her what was at stake. If the school knew that I'd been wagging, we were both in strife – it made her the mentally ill mother who couldn't control her wayward daughter. It was in both of our interests to avoid their scrutiny.

Mum nodded, and sure enough when the principal called she backed me up. The school recommended that I begin seeing the school counsellor. I didn't mind. I got to miss a period of school a week when I met with Miss Meadowcroft. I usually tried to time it so that I missed maths, which I struggled in; I usually spent that period reading. (One day when I had finished a book in class I looked up to see what schoolwork the other students were doing. 'Amra, keep reading,' my maths teacher told me, wanting to avoid my attention-grabbing, classwork-avoiding high jinks.)

'I can't believe that Snežana just ditched me,' I complained to Miss Meadowcroft. 'She said that I was going behind her back and talking about her.'

'Is that what she actually said?'

I frowned, trying to remember. 'Yeah, she said I was talking about her behind her back.'

'Wasn't she angry that you hadn't respected her privacy?' Miss Meadowcroft asked.

I realised that she'd heard Snežana's version because she was also a frequent visitor to the counsellor's office. 'That's not true,' I snapped.

'Did you tell your friends about her home circumstances?'

'I told them that she lived on her own.'

'Do you see how she could be upset about this?' Miss Meadowcroft asked gently.

'No, because it's true. I didn't tell anyone any lies about her.'

Miss sighed and shifted in her chair. 'How would you feel if a friend you trusted told everyone about your home circumstances?'

'What do you mean? That my mum has nervous breakdowns and ends up in hospital? It's the truth. It's what happens.'

I was used to everyone knowing about my life. The Bosnian community was small and we were notorious within it. As soon as people knew the names of my parents they were able to place me, and I would see them finding me wanting. I would pre-empt the judgement of those outside the community by telling them all the sordid details of my life before they had the chance to witness Mum's bizarre behaviour. I didn't see any of this as private, because I was constantly living it publicly.

'Perhaps you and Snežana need to talk about what is private and what is personal,' Miss Meadowcroft said. 'Would you like me to mediate a meeting between the two of you to resolve your issues?'

'There's no point. She ditched me and we're done.'

'Are you sure you want to take such a strong stand?' she asked. 'From what I observed, the two of you were close friends and have a lot in common.'

'I thought so too, but I was wrong. We're not friends anymore. We're nothing.'

After a lifetime of upheaval – having to leave friends, homes and belongings behind in a haphazard fashion when Mum's illness imploded my life – I had developed an impenetrable shield. I was used to leaving people behind and felt no lingering sentimentality about it. For me it was all black and white: our friendship was over and what we'd had was in the past, not to be thought about again.

'What illness does your mum have?' Miss Meadowcroft asked.

This was the first time that we'd explored Mum's illness. Usually I spent all my time bitching about Mum and the way she'd changed since the Balkan War began. She'd become obsessed with being a proper Muslim, and had even begun to pray five times a day. She had to write out the Sura, prayers, and place them around herself to read until she could recite them by heart. She could never fast because she had to take medication, and Muslim fasting prohibited drinking. Muslims were only permitted to rinse their mouths with water.

It wasn't long before she was demanding that Haris and I go to a *Mejtef* that was being delivered out of a community centre not far from us. I loathed the thought of *Mejtef* and didn't want to go back, but Mum put on the emotional blackmail, and now that we had our extended family here there was extra pressure, and I crumbled, going for a few weeks, until boredom meant that I ended up wagging at the local shopping centre.

I told Miss Meadowcroft what happened when Mum got sick and she was the one who finally helped us to identify the medical term for my mother's illness when she gave me a handout listing the symptoms of manic depression (or what we now call bipolar disorder) – something that wouldn't have happened if I didn't become friends with Snežana.

Snežana never knew that she had inadvertently changed my life. After our doomed friendship she blended back into the crowd. I kept Gore Vidal's book as a reminder of that time of my life. I never re-read it, but *Myra Breckinridge* survived my regular book culls, becoming my one sentimental failing.

After this everything changed. We engaged with health professionals as a family. We learnt to be on guard for my mother's symptoms – insomnia, restlessness, excessive spending – and sought help before she was too far gone. Most importantly, my mother started self-monitoring. She learnt to pay attention to her moods and get help if she was feeling too high or too low. Her hospitalisation stays became less frequent and our lives gained stability. Our fractured relationship healed and once again I became her confidante, and she became mine.

THE RUNAWAY BRIDE

I stood in the middle of the dance floor feeling embarrassed and humiliated. It was my first official foray into the dating world, and I had floundered and failed. I was at a Bosnian dance, a *Zabava*, with my friend Monica. Our parents had been friends for decades and we had fallen into a friendship because we were both odd. I was nineteen years old and since finishing high school I had completed a TAFE course in office administration, bypassing university in part because I was intimidated and also because I didn't know what I wanted to study. I had started working full-time as a receptionist and had bought a car. Even though I lived at home, I established my own independence by paying board.

The *Zabava* was an opportunity for Bosnians to mingle with their fellow nationals, and of course for matchmaking to take place between the new arrivals and the Australian-born. Monica and I had attended a Bosnian disco the night before, and I was at the *Zabava* to meet Edo, a boy I'd met there.

I was wearing a black skirt suit that Zehra had given me when she was clearing out her wardrobe. The skirt was skin tight with a deep slit in the back. The jacket was fitted and I hadn't worn a top underneath, so my breasts peeked over the top of the double-breasted lapels. I had paired the outfit with black heels and stockings, looking the part of a glamorous receptionist.

When I walked in, Edo was at a table with his friends Fikret and Emir. Edo came over and said hello, and after we'd made awkward small talk in Bosnian he quickly retreated back to his friends.

I wasn't alone for long. A young man asked me to dance and after we left the dance floor he asked me for my number. I handed him my card. I had made them myself, buying business card stock and printing them on the printer at work, then carefully cutting out the perforated edges.

Over the course of the night many young men asked me to dance, and I gave each one of them my card when they asked. And then came the humiliation. We were sitting around the table and one of the men realised that another man had my number.

'What, you gave him your card too? I don't want it now,' he said in Bosnian, throwing my business card onto the table with disgust.

A blush heated my cheeks and embarrassment hit me. I had committed a faux pas. Until this moment I was a young woman enjoying her femininity – suddenly he had cast me as a harlot. I took my card back and put it in my handbag. The man next to him handed me my card back too. Monica and I stood, moving away from the table, and I asked her advice. We decided the only way to mitigate my humiliation was to take my all of my business cards back.

'What about him?' Monica asked in English and nodded at Fikret, who was sitting at the table next to us with my business card in front of him. He'd had a chat with his friend Edo and had got his permission to ask my number.

While everyone else was making an effort to chitchat,

he was exuding cold indifference. I watched him tearing a serviette, his gaze resting on the white tablecloth in front of him. Most people had attempted to blend in. The women were overdressed in their best finery – shimmering dresses, or skirt suits like mine – the men mostly wore jeans with a nice shirt. His beaten-up leather aviator jacket and bald head and goatee marked him as different, making him stand out in this sea of conformists.

'You'd better be careful what you say,' he told me and Monica in perfect English. 'I can understand every fucking word.' Most of the new arrivals had a rudimentary understanding of English; Fikret was an anomaly who could speak it almost fluently.

'Give me my card back,' I told him, reaching for it.

'No, it's mine. You gave it to me.' He took the card and put it in his jacket pocket.

I felt annoyance mingled with pride. He still wanted my number, despite the blot on my reputation.

After the *Zabava* the group I was with retreated to Cafe Trevi in Carlton. A boy I had been flirting with all night took the seat on one side of me, while my friend Monica sat on the other. I was making small talk with the boy and periodically checking in with Monica. I turned to say something to Monica and suddenly found Fikret next to me. Later he told me that he had spent the night swapping seats until he reached Monica. Monica had stood her ground and refused to swap seats when he asked, so he started making small talk. Finally he complimented her teeth, freaking her out; desperate to be rid of his attention, she shifted seats and he achieved his goal to sit beside me.

We spent the rest of the night talking. He told me about leaving Sarajevo when the conflict started in Croatia. He'd just completed his compulsory army service and would have been the first one to be called up to fight, so his parents sent him away to live with his uncle in Austria for a few months. Instead, war broke out, and Sarajevo was under siege for four years. Separated from his family, unsure if they were alive or dead, he sought work on the black market so he could send them much needed rations.

He lived as a refugee in Austria for two years, at a time when neo-Nazi gangs were beating up foreigners who came across their path. One day they'd caught sight of a Turkish migrant and laid into him with boots and fists. Fikret was walking home and saw the man on the ground, surrounded by gang members. The Nazis stopped to look at Fikret. Fikret froze, waiting for them to turn on him. To them, Fikret was even worse than the Turkish migrant, who at least had a work visa – Fikret was a refugee living off the government who could not work. The neo-Nazis nodded at Fikret, mistaking him for a compatriot because of his white skin, blue eyes and shaved head. Fikret continued walking, hearing the grunts of the Turkish man.

He applied for a visa to Australia, where he would have more work opportunities and he could provide for them. He arrived in 1994, one year before the war finally ended. Now it was 1996 and he was saving to return to Bosnia to be with his family.

I told him about growing up in Australia, about my mum's illness and my extended family coming to Australia since the war began. The hours passed easily as we talked. I remember his blue eyes so steady as they looked into mine. We didn't realise that the table had emptied and everyone had left, until we looked up and saw Monica looking forlorn, sitting by herself at the end of the table.

'I'll walk you to your car.' He stood and offered me his arm. I wound my arm in his and we walked out side by side, Monica following.

As we walked down the street a young man checked me out and I smiled at him. Fikret noticed. 'When we're married you won't be looking at other men,' he said, patting my arm, and I flushed with pride.

He held my car door and I reluctantly got in. 'I'll call you,' he said as he closed the door.

I tracked him in the rear-view mirror as he stood on the street with his hands in his jacket pockets watching me drive away.

'Do you think he'll call me?' I asked Monica.

'Do you want him to? He's so rude.'

'I liked it. He tells it like it is.'

'That's for sure.'

'Listen, I won't sleep over tonight.' I'd packed my bag and had it in the boot. I'd slept over at her house many times before, and we would usually spend most of the next day lazing about together, but I didn't want to miss Fikret calling me.

'Whatever you want.' She sullenly stared out the window and we didn't speak for the rest of the trip.

I dropped her off and drove home. Mum woke up as I unlocked the door, and greeted me in the hallway. 'I thought you were sleeping over at Monica's?'

'I met a boy,' I told her, taking off my high heels with relief. I rubbed the soles of my sore feet. 'His name is Fikret.'

'Really?' Mum's face lit up.

This is what she'd been hoping for. I had dated in the past, but not Bosnian or Muslim boys. I refused to conform to the pressure my family had been putting on me since the war. I made it a point to never let my mother get her hopes up.

I struggled to fall asleep, thinking about all that had happened that night. The next morning I woke up late. After breakfast I lay on the coach, lethargic, within sight of the telephone stand. The phone rang and I stirred, quickly running to answer it. It was Veronica.

'How did it go with Edo?'

'He didn't work out, but I met a guy. His name is Fikret and he's amazing. I'm waiting for him to call, so I have to keep the phone line free.'

'Okay, call me when you hear from him.'

The phone rang again an hour later. It was my grandmother.

'Hello, Nana. I had a really good time at the *Zabava* last night. I met someone,' I said, twirling the phone cord around my finger. 'His name is Fikret. Yes, Mum is here.'

I told Mum, 'Don't talk for long,' as I handed her the phone and returned to the couch.

Mum spoke to Nana quickly, and then we sat on the couch together and watched television.

At two o'clock the phone rang again. 'Oh, Veronica, yeah. He hasn't called yet. Yeah, I'm waiting.' I hung up and lay back down on the couch, feeling teary. He wasn't going to call. Mum had run in from the kitchen, and she looked even more disappointed than me when she realised it wasn't Fikret.

When the phone rang at three o'clock I took my time answering.

'Can I please speak to Amra?' a male voice said, and I straightened up as I recognised Fikret's voice.

'It's me.'

'Great.' He cleared his throat. 'Do you want to go for a coffee at Highpoint?'

'Yes,' I practically squealed.

'Really?' he said, surprise in his voice. He told me later he'd been sure I would say no.

'Where do you want to meet?' I asked.

'I'll pick you up.'

'I can meet you.'

'No, no. I'll pick you up. What's your address?' He said he'd be there by five.

I put on make-up and brushed my hair. I didn't want to overdress for our first date and make it seem like I cared too much, so I put on jeans and a jumper. It was July and a cold winter's night.

'We'd better make coffee,' Mum said when I sat on the couch to wait for Fikret.

'What do you mean?' I switched between channels, keeping an eye on the clock.

'When he comes we have to invite him inside for coffee,' Mum said. 'So we'd better prepare everything.'

'He's not going to come inside,' I said, my voice full of scorn. 'He's going to take me out for coffee.'

'Of course he's going to come inside,' Mum said. 'He's a Bosnian man. He will want to meet your parents.'

I looked at her doubtfully, before reluctantly following her into the kitchen. Perhaps Mum was right. I had never dated a Bosnian man before. Mum prepared a tray with *fildžani* while

I counted out the spoons of coffee into the coffeepot and got the sugar bowl ready. After we finished I waited in the living room, peering through the curtain every few minutes. When the car came up the driveway I squealed and ran to the door.

I could see Mum's look of confusion when she saw Fikret was wearing a denim jacket, his head was clean-shaven and his beard was neatly trimmed. Had she had expected a three-piece suit and tie?

'Would you like to come in?' Mum asked after I had introduced them.

'No, thank you,' Fikret said. 'We're going to go to Highpoint for coffee.'

I put on my shoes and ran for the door, shooting a look of triumph over my shoulder. Mum was left confused. She had thought that a Bosnian man would want to meet the family, but he had behaved with complete disregard for the protocols she had expected. Like most migrants, Mum's cultural expectations had been formed by the homeland she had left behind. In the twenty years since, Bosnia had progressed and so had dating customs, letting young people to establish their own relationships before introducing family to the mix. I was relieved that even though Fikret was Bosnian, he was still his own man.

We went to a cafe in Highpoint and talked, and then he drove me home, parking a few streets away from my parents' house. We made out in the car until my thighs trembled from battling the gearbox between the front seats as the windows steamed up. After Fikret dropped me off at home, I stood in the driveway, the headlights shining on me, and a little devil teased me. I turned my back, bent over and mooned Fikret.

His foot hit the brake and the car jerked when he noticed. I laughed and ran into the house.

He called me when I got home, admonishing me for teasing him, and told me what he wanted us to do together. I told him I was a virgin. I heard the disbelief in his voice and years later he told me that he hadn't believed me. After all, I was a huge flirt and had had boyfriends, but while I'd kissed many a frog, I'd never sealed the deal.

Growing up with a mother who was very forthright about her sexual history had demystified the whole experience, so I didn't find the thought of having sex with any of the sweaty adolescent boys at my high school appealing. My resolve had only been strengthened as I'd observed my high school friends' forays into sexual intercourse, which were characterised by emotional blackmail from horny adolescent boys, and bitter disappointment with the act itself. I made a vow: I would only have sex with my husband. In the meantime, my Mills and Boons were like a horny girl's version of *Playboy* magazine and I spent many hours locked in my bedroom, flicking through the sex scenes, until the pages of my favourite romance novels had curling corners. Now that I was with Fikret, sex seemed like a natural step to take. While he wasn't my husband, he had made his intentions known that he would be one day, and I took him at his word.

The following Saturday I slept over at Fikret's flat and he learnt firsthand that I'd been telling the truth. I came home on Sunday morning and slept till the afternoon. When I woke up at two o'clock Mum told me there was *mutuša* in the oven. I served myself and ate in the kitchen. Mum came in and started washing the dishes. 'How was your date last night?'

'Good.' I hesitated, not sure whether to continue, but Mum was the only one who would be able to help me. 'We tried to do it last night, but it hurt so we stopped.' We had used condoms and hadn't discovered the benefits of external lubricant, and so every time we tried intercourse I had winced at the chafing and he'd immediately stopped. We'd spent the night finding pleasure in other ways, and even though I wasn't a virgin anymore, I somehow felt like a fraud because we hadn't committed the full act.

'It's supposed to hurt,' Mum said. 'You just have to take it.'

'I don't think so.' I threw my spoon on the table 'Why should I take it?'

'Because that's what women do.'

'Maybe that's what you did, but I won't.'

I stormed off to my room and didn't speak to Mum about my sex life again. The next weekend we bought lubricant and all was right with the world.

Two months after we met I told Mum we had decided to move in together. I'd been spending every weekend with Fikret, and the nights that we weren't together we would talk on the phone for hours. We were in a love bubble and completely self-absorbed. It made sense for us to move in together and cut out the commute. Mum was befuddled. She had expected a proposal and a wedding, not for us to 'shack up like Aussies'.

I was also tired of all the drama at home. I was an adult with a job and independence, but Mum was constantly attempting to give me advice me on the proper protocol of courtship. I threw my clothes into a black plastic rubbish bag and drove to Fikret's house. That weekend we returned with a trailer to collect my furniture and the rest of my belongings.

After I'd moved out we travelled up the Calder Freeway from Thornbury to St Albans every weekend to visit my parents. One day my friend Julie called just as we were leaving, and I told her I'd call her back from my parents' phone.

'Don't talk to her too long and leave me alone with your parents,' Fikret admonished me as I drove, knowing my habit of gasbagging with girlfriends for hours.

'I won't. I'll tell her my fiancé is giving me dirty looks.'

'I'm not your fiancé,' he said.

'What? You said we were getting married.'

'When?' He looked confused.

'The first night we met.'

'Yeah, but I was just flirting.'

'Were you?' My foot hit the pedal. We were driving down a steep dip in the road where the speed limit was eighty kilometres an hour. There were no cars in front of us. The needle hovered over the eighty mark, sharply jumped over ninety and settled on 110 as my foot stomped on the gas pedal.

'Slow down,' Fikret screamed, clutching the door handle, his voice high-pitched.

'You can't tell me what to do. You're not my fiancé.'

We arrived at Mum's and spent an awkward night engaging in small talk as we covered over the frosty silence between us.

'I'm sorry about what I said,' he told me as we drove back down that same dip in the road on our way home. 'I want to be your fiancé.'

'I want a ring.'

'We'll go to the jeweller's tomorrow.'

I smiled.

We married eight months after we met. My friends could

not understand why I was getting married so young, and many assumed that I was pregnant. I think my young life of turbulence and constant change had made me long for some certainty. We didn't want to spend our money on an elaborate wedding that neither of us cared about, so instead we had an extended honeymoon in Bosnia with his family.

We hired a wedding dress and a wedding suit and I carried yellow carnations wrapped with a ribbon as my bouquet. We drove ourselves to the wedding together from our one-bedroom flat in Thornbury.

Mum wanted a *Hodža* to marry us in a mosque, followed by a reception. Instead, we had a marriage celebrant and a non-denominational ceremony in Fitzroy Gardens. There was juice and cake from the Cheesecake Shop for the twenty invited guests. Our wedding was intimate and individual. My mother finally got her chance at a fantasy ethnic wedding with proper religious rituals when my brother married Munira, a Bosnian woman in 2008.

I had fought so hard to be the rebel and the black sheep, yet somehow I ended up as part of the flock. At one point the irony bothered me – I had not sought a Bosnian husband; instead, I married a man who happened to be Bosnian – but now I am glad that my mother's wish came true. Her life had been one of turbulence, pain and disapproval, but in the end she triumphed. Her children are her legacy, her vindication and her life's work.

EPILOGUE – 2018

I was watching television, brain dead after a day of teaching, when my home phone rang. I stayed on the couch as Fikret answered. 'It's your brother,' he said, handing me the phone.

Haris had been over on the weekend, a few days before, with Munira, and my niece and nephew. Together with my daughter, Sofia, the three blond-haired children had squealed with happiness as they played hide-and-seek throughout the house, while the adults mostly spoke English, switching to Bosnian when we reached topics that we didn't want the kids to know about.

'Hey, buddy,' I answered.

'Hey. How long since you've seen Mum?' he asked.

I thought back. It was the beginning of term, and I'd been flat-out with after-school meetings, lesson plan preparation and excursions. I was juggling so many things, and time had flown by.

'A couple of weeks.'

For ten years I had lived around the corner from Mum's house in a renovator's delight. I would walk over at least once a week to visit, or Mum and Izet would drop by. A few years ago Fikret and I had realised we were not the renovating types, so we bought a new house and moved a ten minute drive away. I had started booking in a fortnightly catch-up with Mum every Thursday so that I wouldn't neglect seeing her, and yet somehow the weeks had passed by so quickly that I hadn't noticed. Now my stomach plunged. What had I missed?

Mum had been fragile the past few years. Since she'd gone into menopause her bipolar had settled and she had been able to manage it by vigilantly taking her medication and regulating her mood through rigorous routine. Each day she prayed five times, meditated twice, and arranged her day around these habits. Then there was her weekly routine: every Tuesday and Friday she attended a Bosnian women's group; she went to the swimming pool every second day, walking laps in the water to help ease the aches from the rheumatoid arthritis that had weakened her pelvis and knees; and once a week she visited her best friend. She clung to her routine like a buoy in the Pacific Ocean, needing it to keep her afloat, and yet last year she had started struggling to leave the house, her routine slowly becoming eroded.

'I'm scared,' she told me. Her eyes looked lifeless. 'It feels so hard to get out of bed and I sometimes think about dying.'

'Mum, you need to talk to the doctor. There's something wrong.'

She'd been going to the same psychiatrist for over twenty years, and had regular appointments with her GP. Between these two professionals she had successfully managed her bipolar and avoided hospitalisation for over fifteen years. This was something new. She wasn't experiencing the highs and lows of bipolar; instead, she said her body felt heavy and it was like she was rusting from the inside. She told her GP and her psychiatrist, but nothing happened. It was only when her psychiatrist retired and she was allocated a new one through the mental health service that a proper investigation was conducted.

The new psychiatrist ordered a blood test, and the result immediately confirmed the diagnosis. Mum was suffering lithium poisoning. She was supposed to be getting blood tests every three months to ensure that the lithium in her system did not reach toxic levels. Her GP and her psychiatrist had missed it. Her new psychiatrist ordered further tests. A MRI confirmed cysts on her liver and kidney which meant their functioning was being compromised, and she had an enlarged thyroid. And yet despite all her health issues, her sense of humour was undaunted. Last time we spoke she joked: 'I'm a very special person. Now I have a knee specialist, a thyroid specialist, a kidney and liver specialist, and a psychiatrist.'

Now as I waited for my brother respond, I wondered which of her health issues had taken centre stage.

'I think you should go see her,' Haris said. 'Izet has been unwell and she's a bit down.'

My stepfather had had a heart attack ten years earlier, and had been suffering from ill health ever since. His strength and stamina were not what they used to be, and he was constantly complaining of weakness and malaise. He had become a regular visitor to the hospital's emergency department when his chest tightened and he couldn't breathe, but so far there had been no diagnosis. We had started thinking that his symptoms were anxiety induced. After his heart attack and subsequent quadruple bypass we'd received a booklet about possible risk factors that cause heart attacks. My stepfather's blood pressure and cholesterol had been perfect – he'd been a body builder in his youth and had stayed fit throughout his life by exercising every day. He didn't smoke, he wasn't overweight, and he was active. Only one of the risk factors applied to him: isolation and depression.

Izet had always struggled maintaining connections with adults. He'd had a fractured family life and had difficulty trusting people. When they disappointed him, he purged them from his life and never looked back. His only social outlet was visiting coffee shops, and he didn't have any close friends of his own. My stepfather was much more vocal about his health issues and this negatively affected Mum, leaving her exhausted and down.

I called Mum, arranging to visit her that Thursday. Our routine was that I would pick her up and take her to do some clothes shopping, and then we'd eat at a cafe. My stepfather did all the errands and grocery shopping, but he had no patience for chauffeuring Mum so she could shop.

After work I detoured home to pick up Sofia and continued on my way to Mum's.

'Mum, there was such drama today. Boy and girl drama,' Sofia told me as I drove, her voice animated. She was nine years old and we had an after-school ritual of telling each other about our days. I told her about my cheeky students and how I dealt with them, while she told me all about her schoolgirl adventures.

'I found out for sure that my crush Xavier likes me. And Cherie found out her crush doesn't like her, but he likes Emily. And Cherie went crazy. She was chasing everyone all day.'

Grade Four had been characterised by crushes. All the girls obsessed about was who they had a crush on and whether the boys they liked liked them back.

'Why were you running away from Cherie?' I asked.

'Cherie was crazy. She was hitting, punching.' Sofia demonstrated by kicking and punching from the passenger seat.

'Nothing like a girl scorned, huh?' I laughed, keeping my eyes on the traffic in front of us.

'Don't tell Nana and Dido about my crush.'

'Okay, what can we talk about then? We can talk about your swimming.' Sofia had been taking lessons since she was ten months old and was now in the swimming squad. She was working towards a goal of doing forty laps in under twenty-three minutes. 'And we can tell them about your Anzac Day performance.' Sofia had developed her love of guitar because of Izet. A self-taught player, he'd play for her when she was little. He bought her her first guitar when she was four years old, an adult guitar as big as she was. She'd been taking lessons for the past three years and had auditioned for the school band.

'Okay.' Sofia nodded.

We arrived at Mum's. Izet had been slowly renovating the house for the past twenty-five years. In the past ten years he started on the kitchen my father built. Since his heart attack he'd struggled to get back to work on it. My brother had taken over a few months ago, knocking down a wall and installing kitchen cabinets, but he'd been overruled when it came to the plastering. Izet had his preferred specifications and wasn't going to lower his standards, so he had taken over once again and had replaced the studs, installed the insulation, and was slowly putting up the plaster sheets, hindered by his ill health. At least my mother finally had a functional kitchen after ten years with cupboards that had no doors, and a stove with a broken oven.

We arrived and went into the living room. The couch was in the middle, away from the unplastered walls.

'Let's just stay here,' Mum said, looking tired. 'I'll make you dinner. Do you want *pura*?'

Pura was a Bosnian polenta meal, and Mum's speciality.

'That's okay. Fikret made me dinner and it's waiting at home.'

I didn't want her to fatigue herself. Her vertigo was troubling her again and she'd had a hard couple of days where she couldn't move much.

After small talk we got onto the topic of *Bachelor of Paradise*. We discussed the highlights of the show and our favourite couples. Mum had missed some episodes because of her evening prayers, but Izet was an atheist and had watched every one.

There was a lull in the conversation.

'Today at school there were boy dramas and girl dramas,' Sofia told her grandparents.

'What dramas?' I asked, taking on the role of interviewer.

Sofia told them about her crushes, and the discoveries about who liked who.

'I think Xavier likes me,' she ended. 'I always catch him looking at me.'

'You're boy crazy just like your nana.' Mum laughed.

'You were married three times,' Sofia said.

'And lots of boyfriends in between.' Mum slapped her thigh as she laughed, and we all joined her.

'I'll tell you the secret you need to know about boys,' Mum said.

Sofia leaned in and listened.

'You always have to have a replacement ready.'

'That's right. She's been married to Dido for thirty years, but she still might replace him.' I pointed at my laughing stepfather. 'He'll just have to wait and see.'

'Your mum wasn't boy crazy like your nana,' Mum said, looking at me.

'Yes, she was. She stalked her crushes,' Sofia said.

I had told Sofia about Dragon, my Year Seven crush. I realised that my mother and I had spent most of my adolescence estranged. She had told me her stories, but I had never told her mine.

'Maybe you're more like me than I thought,' Mum said, looking at me.

'Maybe I am.'

While there had been years of tension in our relationship as I struggled to accept my mother's illness and the effect it had on her, my daughter was helping us bridge the gap.

The next day Sofia pulled me aside. 'I've been thinking. I think that Allen can be my back-up,' she said.

I laughed. 'Your grandmother will be so proud when I tell her.'

ACKNOWLEDGEMENTS

This book took five years to write, and a lifetime to gestate. There are many people who I need to thank for their generosity of spirit and practical advice.

My mother Fatima – while it was an accident of biology that you birthed me, it was your love and care that made me who I am. You were generous with your stories and with my requests for interviews and clarifications. Writing this book has been the hardest thing I've ever done and you eased my fears after reading my first draft when you called me and said: 'you really love me,' and 'you know me the best out of anyone.' Yes, and yes.

My husband Fikret has been my first reader, my therapist, and my cheerleader. Thank you for being my sounding board and for believing in me when I didn't believe in myself.

My daughter Sofia, you are the love of my life and you make every day sparkle with laughter.

My grandmother Adevija – while you have been gone for six years, you are always with me.

My great-grandmother Muradija – for gifting the women in our family with the storytelling gene.

Thank you to the rest of my family for being my support system and fountain of inspiration.

Veronica Ho and Jodi Wiley for your friendship and the conversations that always lift me up.

Alice Pung for being my mentor and helping me to find the time and motivation to write the first draft. Your unwavering belief in this memoir being published is what prodded me to try, try and try again.

Creative Victoria for funding my mentorship and professional development to complete my first draft.

Barry Scott for believing in my book, Penelope Goodes for your editorial suggestions, and everyone at Transit Lounge for being a part of my team.

My writing group Pink Ladies – Christine Mackley, Renee Robinson, Phelon Manski – for helping to keep me motivated, for reading my drafts and giving me great suggestions and critiques.

My other writing group Destineers for being a wonderful network of strong women.

Simmone Howell for reading an early draft and helping me realise the strength of my story.

Amy Barker for your encouragement and critique on extracts that were published along the way.

Pippa Masson for your suggestions and advice.

My year 10 Creative Writing students for reading my prologue and being suitably impressed their teacher is a writer, and Kellie Phan for being a kindred spirit who is a passionate young adult reader.

Writing a book is a hard journey and finding confidence to keep going is sometimes difficult to discover. It is the small kernels of hope offered by anthology and journal editors who published extracts that helped me on my journey. *Meet Me at the Intersection* editors Ambelin Kwaymullina and Rebecca Lim, *Rebellious Daughters* editors Lee Kofman and Maria

Katsonis, and *Etchings Journal* publishers Sabina Hopfer and Christopher Lappas, and editor Amy Nicholls-Diver.

And thank you also to the members of my writing community who encouraged me when I was flailing about the many years it took to write this book.

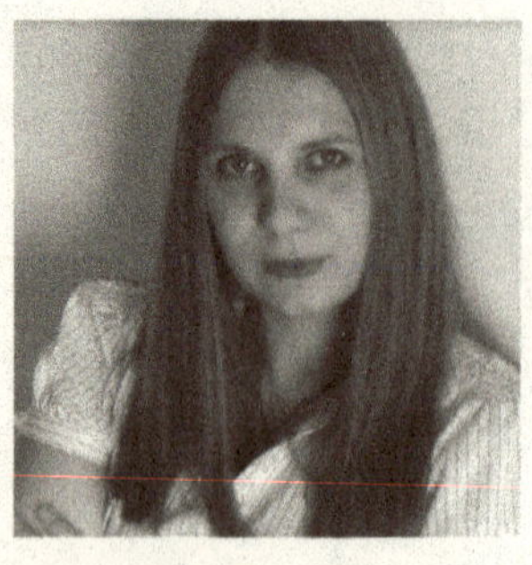

Amra Pajalić is a Melbourne-based author of Bosnian background. Her debut novel *The Good Daughter* (Text Publishing, 2009) won the 2009 Melbourne Prize for Literature's Civic Choice Award, and was a finalist in the 2009 Melbourne Prize for Literature Best Writing Award. Prior to publication it was shortlisted in the 2007 Victorian Premier's Awards for Best Unpublished Manuscript. She is also author of a novel for children, *Amir: Friend on Loan* (Garratt Publishing, 2014).

Amra is co-editor of the anthology *Growing up Muslim in Australia* (Allen and Unwin, 2018) that was shortlisted for the 2015 Children's Book Council of Australia Eve Pownall Award for Information Books. She also wrote the teaching notes published by Allen and Unwin.

Amra has appeared on panels at conferences and literary festivals including at the Wheeler Centre, Melbourne Writers Festival, Williamstown Literary Festival, Reading Matters Conference Panel, and the VicTESOL Conference. She has delivered workshops and presented at various library and community organisations, and was a judge and convenor of the Premier's Awards for an Unpublished Manuscript.

She was funded by Artists in Schools to be an Artist in Residence in 2010, 2011 and 2012 in high schools, and in 2014 received funding from Creative Victoria to be mentored by Alice Pung to work on her memoir.

She works as a high school teacher and is completing a PhD in Creative Writing at La Trobe University. Her website is www.amrapajalic.com.